ROOO41 53499

D1509239

PARENTS AS
LANGUAGE THERAPISTS

To the parents and their children
who participated in this project.

PARENTS AS LANGUAGE THERAPISTS

Second Edition

Roger J. Rees, B.Sc. (Hons), M.Ed., Ph.D.
South Australian College of Advanced Education

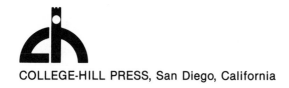

COLLEGE-HILL PRESS, San Diego, California

Second Edition

College–Hill Press, Inc.
4284 41st Street
San Diego, California 92105

© 1984 by College–Hill Press

All rights, including that of translation, reserved. No part of this publication may be reproduced, stored in a retrieval system, or transmitted in any form or by any means, electronic, mechanical, recording, or otherwise, without the prior written permission of the publisher.

Library of Congress Cataloging in Publication Data

Rees, Roger J.
    Parents as language therapists.

    "A final report for the National Advisory Council for the Handicapped, Department of Social Security, and the Inger Rice Trust."

    Bibliography: p.
    Includes indexes.
    1. Speech disorders in children. 2. Mentally handicapped children—Education—Language arts. 3. Speech therapy. 4. Domestic education.
I. National Advisory Council for the Handicapped (Australia) Dept. of Social Security. II. Inger Rice Trust. III. Title.
RJ496.S7R44   1984   618.92'855   84-15588

ISBN 0-933014-49-X

Printed in the United States of America

100252 1

Acknowledgements

This longitudinal research would not have been possible without the generous supporting grants from the Inger Rice Foundation, and the National Advisory Council for the Handicapped, Department of Social Security. A further generous grant from an anonymous Melbourne donor greatly helped with the employment of additional personnel.

The regular use of facilities in the School of Education at the Canberra College of Advanced Education, the Capital Territory Health Commission clinics and the A.C.T. Schools Authority Special Schools were vital in this research. I am grateful for the easy access to these facilities. I am grateful to my many colleagues in the School of Education and in particular to Max Kemp, to the staff of the Capital Territory Health Commission and the A.C.T. Schools Authority who have given me so much support and help during this time.

Research of this nature involved many people with particular educational, social, psychological and medical expertise. I am particularly grateful to Dr. M. G. Williams, Director of Health Services at Canberra C.A.E., for his quiet encouragement and advice, to Professor G. M. Kneebone, Department of Pediatrics, School of Medicine, Flinders University, S.A., for his examination of a cross section of children participating in the programme and to Professor R. D. Strom, Arizona State University, U.S.A., for his advice and help in the evaluation of parents' attitudes to teaching their children.

Parents of the intellectually handicapped in the A.C.T. and district attended lectures and seminars on the effectiveness of intervention programmes for the intellectually handicapped given by Professor A. D. B. Clarke and Dr. A. M. Clarke from the University of Hull, U.K. This led parents with intellectually handicapped children to request and play a part in establishing the intervention programme described in this report. In the meetings prior to the establishment of this research, there were many difficulties and little cohesion. However, the unflagging support and skill of Dr. J. W. Irvine and Professor Don Fitzgerald of the Centre for Behavioural Studies, University of New England, Armidale, N.S.W., enabled this research to maintain its momentum in a realistic and controlled form.

Research of this nature depends so much on the vigour and enthusiasm of all those participating. In particular, Dr. Irvine and Mrs. Kaye Pickering, Speech Therapist with the Capital Territory Health Commission, played vital roles. Dr. Irvine's persistent reminders of the need to attend to the fine details of this research were always presented in a most acceptable form. His friendship and skill throughout these years were vital. The Language Manual written for use in this programme is integral to the parent training. Kaye Pickering's participation in the writing of the Manual and her skill in teaching from it set such a fine example to all the other professionals involved. This programme would have been impossible without her teaching skill and capacity to understand the needs of the families of the intellectually handicapped. I owe a particular debt of gratitude to her. The support of my wife Deborah and the skill of Jan Wotton in proof reading and preparing the index are also most gratefully acknowledged.

Finally, to the parents and their children who participated during these years, I am grateful for the pleasure of having worked with them, for their openness to enquiry, and for the numerous examples of their ability to withstand demanding teaching and interpersonal situations with such fine humour and good spirit.

Abstract

One hundred and thirty five families with moderate and severely intellectually handicapped children established a language training programme for their handicapped children. One hundred and two families and their children (Mean C A 5 years 8 mths at the commencement of the programme) stayed involved for the programme's thirty three months duration. The programme was in three stages. Stage I, which lasted for one year, was a year of preparation. At the end of this year a sequential criterion referenced language teaching manual was produced for use during Stages II and III. Parents contributed to the preparation of this manual. Stage II lasted for nine months. During this time four different methods of intervention were trialled and evaluated. At the beginning of this stage, the children and their families were divided into four groups: A, B, C and D. Group A received the language manual, group training for parents in behaviour modification techniques and weekly behaviour modification techniques for the children on an individual basis. This method of intervention, known in the programme as Target Teaching, lasted for the full nine months. Group B received the language manual, group discussions with social workers and individual home visits from the social workers. This method of Social Work/Supportive Counselling lasted for six months, thereafter Group B received the Target Teaching programme for three months. Group C received the language manual, group training for parents in speech therapy techniques and weekly speech therapy for the children on an individual basis. This method of Speech Therapy training lasted for six months, thereafter Group C received the Target Teaching programme for three months. Group D received only the language manual and no other means of intervention. This method for Group D (known as Language Programme only) lasted for the full nine months of Stage II. Stage III, which lasted for one year was a year of follow up. The Stage III programme was common for all families. They received group help and advice and where necessary, speech therapy for their children on an individual basis. The programme was evaluated by using the Reynell Developmental Language Scales (Reynell 1969b), to assess the children's receptive and expressive language skills. This took place at the beginning and end of Stage I, at the end of each three month period during Stage II and again at the end of Stage III. A sample of children had their IQ levels assessed at the beginning and end of the programme by the Stanford Binet (Form LM) IQ test (Terman & Merrill 1961). Parents of the children responded at the commencement of Stage II to an individual inventory (Strom & Slaughter 1976) to evaluate their attitudes towards teaching their intellectually handicapped children. Each week for thirty weeks during Stage II, all children's receptive and expressive language skills were assessed on the criterion referenced tasks that they were being taught. Weekly records were kept by parents of their language teaching, for examination and instructional purposes during group training sessions. A selection of parents teaching their children criterion referenced tasks from the language manual were videotaped for instructional purposes during group training sessions. Multivariate analysis of covariance (MANCOVA) or multivariate analysis of variance (MANOVA) was used to analyse the children's receptive and expressive language age scores and to determine any significant differences in group scores. Pearson product moment correlation coefficients were computed to analyse the reliability of children's IQ scores and the relationship between IQ scores and receptive and expressive language age scores. Results indicated: (i) that Target Teaching was the most effective method for teaching children receptive language skills especially over a short-term period of three months; (ii) that the behaviour modification Target Teaching was superior to the

Language Programme Only; in the teaching of receptive language skills in both the short term period of three months, over nine months and over a period of twenty one months; (iii) that children whose parents received nine months of Target Teaching training during Stage II, were most able to maintain their children's receptive language age score gains during Stage III; (iv) that Target Teaching and Speech Therapy were equally effective in teaching children expressive language skills over the three and six months period; (v) that the Language Programme Only was the least effective method for teaching **both** receptive and expressive language skills particularly when compared with the Target Teaching programme; (vi) that children's sex, etiology and level of language development did not affect their receptive and expressive language performance; (vii) that the children's IQ scores were reliable but should not be regarded as fixed or unchanging; (viii) that there was a closer relationship between children's IQ scores and their receptive language age scores than between children's IQ scores and their expressive language age scores; (ix) that parents' responses to the attitude inventory helped identify their frustration and difficulties in teaching their children and that examination of parent responses indicated those parents who were most and least able to teach their children; (x) that individual criterion referenced case studies indicated the nature of the teaching, the particular difficulties children had with learning receptive and expressive language skills, the number of teaching sessions required to teach children even the simplest skill and the perseverence and ingenuity of the parents and families involved. However, this perseverance and ingenuity was often put at risk by the fragmentation of services for families with intellectually handicapped children. Teachers, Speech Therapists, Occupational Therapists, Counsellors and Social Workers combined for the thirty three months of this project to provide an integrated service. This contributed much to parents staying in the programme, to parents openness to the professionals involved and to parents persistence in teaching their children language skills.

Preface

Over the past decade, the use of non-professionals in dealing with the developmental problems of the intellectually handicapped has greatly increased. These non-professionals include, in particular, volunteer workers and parents. Parents are a focal point of this research. They have been involved for three years in teaching and evaluating their childrens' language skills.

102 families with intellectually handicapped children from the A.C.T., the City of Queanbeyan, and the town of Yass in N.S.W. participated for three years in this language teaching programme. The definitions and categories of moderate and severe intellectual handicap of the subjects are those used by the Assessment Clinic (T.A.C.) of the Capital Territory Health Commission and by the Counselling Service of the A.C.T. Schools Authority. Psychologists, counsellors, teachers and speech therapists employed by the A.C.T. Schools Authority played a vital role in this community based programme. They have been largely responsible for the relatively small number of families withdrawing from the programme.

This report is in three parts. Part One has four chapters. Chapter One identifies the problems of the research and the nature of the sample involved. Chapter Two is a review of the literature in which critical parent training variables are identified and evaluated. This chapter concludes with a critique of the distinct features of some intervention programmes of the 1970s. Chapter Three presents a rationale for parent involvement and describes the nature and stages of the teaching programmes. Chapter Four describes the assessment procedures, the problems of internal and external validity in longitudinal research and presents the null hypotheses to be tested.

Part Two is concerned with the results of the study. There are three chapters. Chapter Five examines the effectiveness of interventions as indicated by childrens' measured receptive and expressive language skills. It answers questions about the reliability and stability of the IQ scores of the intellectually handicapped and their relationship with language development. The chapter points out the importance of children's IQ score changes in parent motivation. Chapter Six describes the relationship between parents' expressed attitudes and their difficulties and aspirations in teaching their children. Chapter Seven contains five case studies in which an examination of the effectiveness of reinforcement procedures in home based teaching is presented.

Part Three contains one chapter. Chapter Eight presents some answers to the problems of the research raised in Chapter One. It presents general answers to the research questions raised in Chapter Four, and it concludes with identifying areas which clearly require further research.

These research priorities apply to families, schools and clinics who have responsibility for the care, upbringing and above all the language development of the intellectually handicapped.

A three stage *Language Manual* written for use in the Parents as Language Therapists program is available. This is referred to in the abstract and in the Parents as Language Therapists text. It is not included in the appendices to this book.

The 50 page Manual contains: "Preliminary exercises for developing speech," 26 sequenced receptive language exercises and 26 related and sequenced expressive language exercises. The *Language Manual* can be obtained by writing to:

>The Director,
>Institute for the Study of Learning Difficulties,
>Faculty of Health Sciences and Education,
>South Australian College of Advanced Education,
>Sturt Road,
>*BEDFORD PARK. SOUTH AUSTRALIA. 5042.*

The price of the *Language Manual* is $6 Australian, including postage and packing. Please make cheques payable to "Institute for the Study of Learning Difficulties." Payments from countries other than Australia should be by international money order or bank draft.

Contents

CHAPTER SEVEN (Continued) Page

PART THREE — CONCLUSION

CHAPTER EIGHT   CONCLUSIONS AND RECOMMENDATIONS FOR FURTHER RESEARCH

APPENDICES — Used during Research (available from author)

(I)	Samples of Literature Distributed to Parents during Stage 1
(II)	Preparatory, Receptive and Expressive Language Criterion Check Lists*
(III)	The Language Teaching Manual
(IV)	Language Statements Presented to Parents during Stage 1**
(V)	Sample Receptive and Expressive Language Profile Recorded at 0_2
(VI)	Individual Stanford Binet IQ Scores at 0_1 and 0_6
(VII)	Strom's Parent as a Teacher (PAAT) Attitude Inventory
(VIII)	Occupational Classification of Parents
(IX)	Parent as a Teacher Individual Profile
(X)	Reynell Receptive Language Age Scores and Reynell Expressive Language Age Scores Observed Cell Means for Six Periods

*See page 227.
**See page 233.

TABLES

FIGURES

PART ONE

THE RESEARCH PROBLEMS AND ISSUES

Chapter One

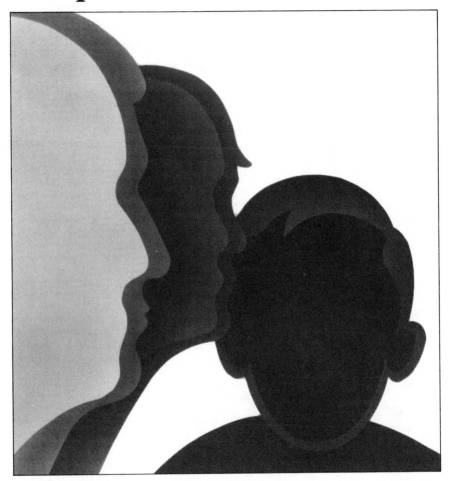

The Nature of the Problem and Sample

INTRODUCTION

Improving expectations for intellectually handicapped children and developing concepts of normalization have aided parents in their decision as to whether to keep these children at home or to institutionalize them. The result is that the great majority of families do keep their children at home, certainly during their formative years. This is a general description but holds true for the families with intellectually handicapped children who live in the Australian Capital Territory, the City of Queanbeyan, and the Town of Yass.

For a variety of different reasons that are not yet wholly comprehended, at least one in every hundred children is born intellectually handicapped. Many others become so during the early months or years of life due to illness or injury. Some of these are mildly handicapped. Yet very many, like the children described in this research, are moderately or, more particularly, severely intellectually handicapped. In many cases these children have additional associated handicaps and, as such, will have to be looked after for the rest of their lives. These children are spending their childhood years at home living with their families.

This research is about such families — families in which a child of the family is intellectually handicapped. The research describes how the parents endeavoured to teach their children communication and language skills. These are ordinary families — not in any condescending sense of being uninteresting or greatly alike, but in being little different from the people next door or the family in another suburb who do not happen to have an intellectually handicapped child. This needs to be stressed because the research revealed that often among other parents, and indeed professionals, there is a tendency to treat families with an intellectually handicapped child as somehow different.

For all of these families the birth of a non-handicapped child was hoped for and anticipated. Adjustments have had to be made to cope with the intellectually handicapped child. In part, this is because their future is uncertain. Indeed, for many families the future is often clouded with doubts. Expectations for the intellectually handicapped are improving. Yet social stigma still exists and there are various misconceptions abroad about anyone who keeps a severely intellectually handicapped child at home. Parents of these children often fear the future and are super-cautious about the present. After all, as one mother put it, "there's an adage abroad that a handicapped child makes a handicapped family". To feel different is to feel isolated and alone. Defensiveness pervades. In this atmosphere initiative and enthusiasm can seep away. Then only the more resolute are able to persist with teaching their children skills and with planning for attainment of identifiable goals based on models of physical, social and linguistic normality.

It was in pursuit of these goals that a group of parents of intellectually handicapped children from the Australian Capital Territory, the city of Queanbeyan and the town of Yass, requested the Capital Territory Health Commission to provide improved speech therapy services for their children. Like others before them, these parents felt that tackling their children's speech problems would be likely to help social interaction and remove much of the stigma associated with the poor communication skills of the intellectually handicapped. This is the key problem of this research. The children's intellectual retardation has hindered their social interaction, or more specifically, the quite delayed receptive and expressive language skills have meant that social interaction was almost impossible. Therefore, if the children's receptive and expressive language skills could be improved by effective teaching, would improved social interaction in the home and elsewhere follow?

It was, and is, important for these parents to be able to maintain a realistic hope. In this setting they are able to make meaningful demands on their children. Without this realistic hope, appropriate teaching could, and would, be abandoned. As such, the parents may come to expect less of their children than they are capable of accomplishing.

Reasons for Parental Involvement

Why did these parents become involved in establishing their own language intervention programme? "To help my child to talk" was a standard answer. But really the reasons are deeper than this. Indeed, they must have been (in part at least) for parents to sustain their home-based teaching and also their attendance at group meetings and individual clinic sessions for the three years of this project. It may appear as something of a surprise to hear some parents remark that "achieving justice for my child" was a stated reason. But a balanced sense of justice may be regarded as so much a part of the social and biological equipment of man. For other parents it was an appreciation of the plasticity of the child and of the extent to which this could be used by effective teaching. For others there was a belief that if their child could talk, closer approximation to normality would develop. Thus, both the emotions and the intellect of these parents led them to request, to establish and to participate in this intervention programme.

Initial Identification of Tasks and Goals

At the outset of this programme no-one knew the form it would take. No-one knew whether parents would really become involved or for how long they and the professionals would persist. To begin with, three major tasks had to be undertaken:
  (i) to find out about the nature of the sample population of children and to spend time with families assessing the children and examining the nature and degree of parent and professional involvement that was both desirable and possible;
 (ii) to design a language programme which utilized existing "helping" agencies already involved with these parents and their children, and to design a programme which took account of current research in language acquisition;
(iii) to establish a programme which comprehensively evaluated both the language gains made by the children and the influence of parent variables such as their attitudes and skills.

Parents' Adjustment and Co-operation

Initially no funds for the project existed and the parents had to hope that funds would become available. It is sometimes difficult for those with minimal knowledge of families with handicapped children to realise that these parents believed in the uniqueness of their children and took a great pride in the skills, however meagre, that these children possessed. Yet however confidently these parents have talked of treating the children as normal and ensuring that "he is just another member of the family group", throughout they have had to make changes in their way of life to fit it comfortably around the handicapped member.

It was not the business of an intervention programme such as this to take over domestic routines nor to control a child's every movement, but rather to encourage parents' efforts and develop and utilize parents' imagination. It became evident that, no matter what the cause and degree of retardation, a collaborative effort with parents was an essential part of the undertaking. Furthermore, as the project evolved, parents and professionals not only advanced their own clinical knowledge but increased their circle of friends from among those involved in the project and their intimacy with specific friends. This face to face social network was vital in helping parents and professionals **sustain** their efforts during these three years.

Parents' Aspirations

In many cases the examination of this sample of families with intellectually handicapped children has shown that they have had high expectations for their children and, as such, have found their dreams and aspirations disrupted. They have had to shuffle their plans, reshape relationships, change ambitions, drop hobbies, develop new interests, ideas and friends, and in so many ways become a different unit.

Family Problems

One of the most important factors in the teacher's or therapist's capacity to help these parents is his or her awareness of the extraordinary problems that face families living with a severely intellectually handicapped child. In many ways, nothing short of living with such a child and taking care of him can produce an awareness of the very great wear and tear, both physically

6

and psychologically, that occurs and its reciprocal effect on parent-child relationships. In part, therefore, this research is concerned with how these families cope, adjust and develop. It is concerned with identifying which variables help determine the families that are successful in teaching their children. Religious beliefs, socioeconomic status, educational background, and the presence or absence of extended family and community supports are some of the additional variables that were observed to interact with the severity of the child's disability to influence parental reactions. Thus, while degree of impairment is an important factor, it is difficult, if not impossible, to predict whether parents are able to adjust more adequately to mild or severe problems caused, on the face of it, by having a handicapped child.

Family Endurance Group Cohesion and Professional Responsibility

The day to day problems of caring for the intellectually handicapped child make it very easy for parents to focus on the negative aspects of their lives. This aspect needed to be borne in mind throughout the years of this language intervention programme. Yet this programme demonstrates the endurance, emotional strength, keen humour and persistence of these parents. These factors were important in providing group cohesion and enabling some parents to become obvious leaders in their groups. These "leader" parents in particular were open, pliant and persistent. They made it clear that a warm family and community atmosphere was, for them, the most desirable setting for healthy, normal experiences and optimal development of their intellectually handicapped children. In part, therefore, a responsibility for the professional was to help facilitate this warm, accepting, yet challenging, community atmosphere.

The Children's Language Disabilities

The children in this programme suffer from *severe language* delay. This generally has affected every aspect of development and, of course, can have potentially devastating effects on their educational, emotional and interpersonal development. (One might ask the question whether the retarded educational, emotional and interpersonal development has contributed to the severe language delay. This, of course, is a familiar "chicken and egg" question in language development of the intellectually handicapped). In examining the developmental consequences of the speech and language disabilities of these children, it became readily apparent that language delay and expressive aphasia were interacting factors in the children's educational and cognitive development. This language delay was much more of a handicap than speech disabilities such as articulation or timing problems. This is because the children's educational and cognitive development depend heavily on the understanding and use of language. The educational and cognitive development of these intellectually handicapped children are interactive in nature and do rely on a mutuality between understanding and expressing ideas.

Verbal Comprehension and Expression

Improving the children's understanding and expression was to become the focus of the parent intervention. The parents of these children realised that the absence of linguistic competence obviously hampers such interaction and interferes with optimal cognitive development. Parents were also aware that their children's expressive language delay was associated with delay in non-verbal mental abilities as well as verbal abilities. The nature of these non-verbal and verbal abilities and the relationship between them was to become more fully comprehended by both parents and professionals as the programme progressed.

Sensitivity to Parents

It was important at all stages that the professionals involved in the programme be sensitive to parental responses. It was essential that parents were *not* overwhelmed with too much or too technical information. At the same time, it was necessary that, in their concern for the parents, the professionals should not present a falsely optimistic prognosis. Throughout the programme it was important for the professionals to make allowances for parents' reactions. It was vital for the professionals to avoid biased or prejudical *ad hoc* judgments. Parents' behaviours, and attitudes had to be carefully evaluated. As such, the nature of the programme's problems were:
(i) to have those participating parents involved in *every* stage of the research; that is, to include them in discussions, to allow them to observe language testing and to inform them of the

7

results, to include parental ideas in the production of the language programme so that
-parents could identify closely with the written language programme;

(ii) to produce a realistic plan of teaching which enabled parents to teach on a day-to-day basis. This plan had to take into account the needs of the child, the capacities of family and professional resources;

(iii) to make provision for regular modification or amendment of the programme and to let the parents know that at any time they could suggest and implement modifications;

(iv) to make clear to parents and all participating professionals the resources available for use in such a language intervention programme; to make clear to parents in group meetings how they could use resources made available in the programme;

(v) to include parents, wherever possible, in the regular assessment procedures as well as the actual teaching; to provide opportunities for observation of parent-child interaction and opportunities, both individually and in groups, for parents to discuss the effectiveness of their teaching;

(vi) to teach parents about the distinctive features of language development; to arrange for instructions and for reports to be written in clear, understandable, jargon-free language. It needed to be clearly understood by all the professionals that information about language development that parents did not understand was useless;

(vii) to help parents keep records and share (or have an input) in writing of reports. This enabled parents to realise that there is no such thing as a final, unchanging diagnosis. To encourage the parent to ask for copies of the child's records; to communicate these case histories in terms of data. For instance, that the child was "anxious" or that he "stammered", does not describe the situation nor the level at which the child is operating;

(viii) to encourage the parents to talk freely and openly with many professionals and other parents in individual and group training sessions; to use this parental input to demonstrate that life with the child is part of an ongoing, problem-solving, process in which much attention is given to the child's abilities and assets as well as his or her deficiencies and disabilities;

(ix) to help parents recognise that professionals have distinct roles to play and that from time to time there may be conflicts between different professional groups; to equip parents with advice and skills as to how to make their way through the system of "helping services";

(x) to help parents to stay in close touch with the children's teacher or therapist during the course of the programme and to help all parents to realise that persuasion requires confidence and coolness, and that this is so often based on parents being aware and confident about their own abilities and intuitions; to demonstrate to parents that they should be confident when talking to professionals, remembering that they know the child far better than anyone else.

NATURE OF THE SAMPLE

Chronological Ages and Distribution into Etiology Groups

Parents established the language training programme. Therefore while parents could be advised that the programme might not be suitable for their child, they could not be denied the opportunity of participating once the programme was established. One hundred and thirty-five intellectually handicapped children were pre-tested at the commencement of the programme at 0_1* (see Chapter 3, Figure 3.1 and Chapter 4). During the three years of the programme 33 families either withdrew or moved away from the Australian Capital Territory. The 102 children and their families, referred to in the sample tables, are those who participated in the programme for its three years' duration. The nature of this sample is described in the following tables (1.1, 1.2, 1.3, 1.4 and Fig. 1.1).

* 0_1 refers to the first testing period of the programme.

TABLE 1.1

Mean Chronological Age, Standard Deviation and Age Range
of Total Sample at the Commencement of the Programme

Group	N	\multicolumn{3}{c}{Chronological Age (CA) in Months}
		M	SD	Age Range
Boys	58	72	33	22 to 142
Girls	44	62	33	20 to 139
Total	102	68	31	20 to 142

TABLE 1.2

Etiology and Number of Subjects

Group	Down's Syndrome	Brain Damaged	Epilep- tic	Hydro- cephalic	Micro- cephalic	Genetic Disorder	Other M.H. *
Boys	31	7	3	1	5	4	7
Girls	26	9	2	-	4	-	3
Total	57	16	5	1	9	4	10

* Other Mentally Handicapped refers to moderately and severely Intellectually
Handicapped children whose handicap is due to no known organic origin.

TABLE 1.3

Mean Chronological Age and Standard Deviation in Months
according to Etiology at the Commencement of the Programme

Group	Down's Syndrome		Brain Damaged		Epilep- tic		Hydro- cephalic		Micro- cephalic		Genetic Disorder		Other M.H.	
	M	SD	M	SD	M	SD	M	SD	M	SD	M	SD	M	SD
Boys	66	32	92	40	62	23	54	-	54	12	67	42	101	24
Girls	58	33	62	24	84	19	-	-	59	25	-	-	91	21
Total	63	30	75	32	83	22	54	-	56	18	67	42	98	23

Chronological Ages and IQ Scores for the Sample

Sixty-six children in the sample were tested for general ability at both O_1 and again at the conclusion of the programme at O_6 (see Ch. 3 and Fig. 3.1, p. 54 and Ch. 4, p. 105)*. The individual and group mean IQ scores computed for these children are presented below in Table 1.4. A histogram showing the distribution of individual IQ scores at the commencement of the programme is presented in Figure 1.1, p. 15.

* O_6 refers to the sixth (final) testing period of the programme.

TABLE 1.4

Stanford Binet IQ Scores and Mean Chronological Ages in
Months of Sixty-six Subjects* at the Commencement of the Programme

Group	N	CA M	CA SD	IQ M	IQ SD
All Down's Syndrome	41	74	30	40.4	9.7
All Other	25	89	29	39.4	8.9
Brain Damaged	8	94	30	37.4	5.9
Mentally Handicapped	10	98	23	42.5	11.3
All Boys	43	86	26	38.8	8.6
All Girls	23	70	31	41.8	10.2
Down's Boys	22	80	22	38.0	8.6
Down's Girls	19	64	28	43.1	10.1
Total	66	79	30	39.9	9.4

* The sixty-six children with IQ scores at O_1 (the first phase of testing) are considered to be representative of the total sample. The children excluded were either too young at O_1 (less than 2½ years of age) or were not available for IQ testing at O_1. The children included here are also those children who were still in the programme at O_6 (see Ch. 3 and Fig. 3.1 p. 54). It should be noted that all children are thirty-three months older at the end of the programme O_6 (see Fig. 3.1. p. 54).

These one hundred and two children (see Tables 1.1, 1.2 and 1.3) were taught language and communication skills during the three years of this project (see Chapter 3). These children's language and concept skills were carefully assessed and the results appear in Chapters 5, 6 and 7. It was the children's parents who participated in the programme and who made clear their aspirations, difficulties and attitudes towards teaching their children (see Chapter 6 and 7).

10

FIGURE 1.1

Distribution of Stanford Binet (Form LM) I Q Scores
for the total sample (66 subjects) at O_1 (Mean Chronological
Age 6 years 7months, S.D.: 2 yrs. 6mths.

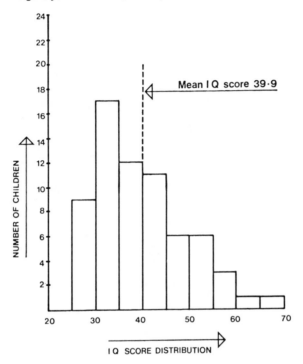

Chapter Two

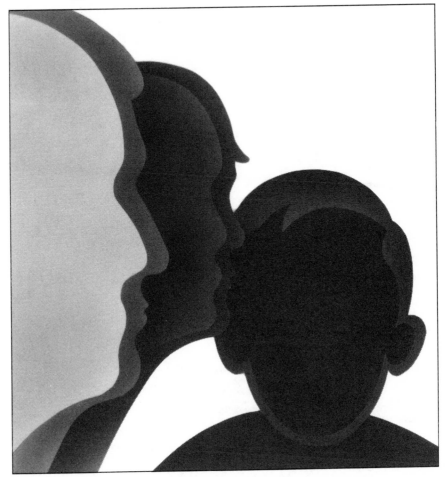

Factors Influencing the Success
of Home Based Language
Intervention Programmes for
Severely Intellectually Handicapped
Children — A Review

SUMMARY

It would be simple to concentrate on the influence of factors such as age, sex, etiology, language level and treatment programmes as factors likely to influence the success of a parent training programme. However, a comprehensive long term parent training programme requires the professionals involved to be aware of and sensitive to a wide range of issues, each of which might affect the outcome, of both parent teaching and children's language acquisition.

This review outlines the growing awareness by parents of their vital role in their intellectually handicapped children's development. It identifies parents' needs, difficulties and aspirations in bringing up an intellectually handicapped child. It comments on variables which might determine the success of a parent oriented intervention programme, on when it should commence, and on the need for professionals to take account of often quite different parent reactions to handling their intellectually handicapped child. It emphasises that parent aspirations for their intellectually handicapped children are similar to the aspirations for their non handicapped children no matter what the age, sex, etiology or language level of the intellectually handicapped child.

In this language intervention programme, the roles of professionals such as speech therapists, teachers, social workers and counsellors, are described. It is then emphasised that currently the great majority of parent intervention programmes are behaviourally oriented. The strategies of behaviour modification may suit short term behavioural objectives. The language problems of the intellectually handicapped child are distinct and there may not be responses from them, at least in the short term, to specific environmental contingencies. It is emphasised that understanding the role of cognition in language development will help to decide both content and goals of language teaching, and probably also teaching methods. Different approaches to teaching language are reviewed and the difficulties that parents may have with operant programmes are identified. Finally, variables, such as parent education, parent attitudes to teaching, the time span of parents' teaching, follow up procedures, and contingency contracting in maintaining parent involvement, are examined as possible determinants of the success of a home based language intervention programme.

EARLY HISTORY

Parental role and expectations for the intellectually handicapped child have changed much in the last twenty years. Indeed, since the establishment of intervention programmes, there have been many reports and writings which emphasise the possible constructive effects of these programmes (Bissell, 1970; Burden, 1977; Clarke and Clarke, 1974; Heber, Dever and Conroy, 1968; Heber et al., 1972; Stanford Research Institute, 1971a and 1971b; Tjossem, 1976; World Health Organisation, 1968). It can also be said that attitudes towards the intellectually handicapped have changed more in the last twenty years than in the preceding two hundred years (Keys Smith, 1975; Kushlick, 1968). Indeed, in the United States of America now, Public Law 94-142, the Education for All Handicapped Children Act, requires that each handicapped child be provided with an individualised written education programme (EIP), the preparation of which must involve the child's parents or guardians. Therefore, in the U.S.A. the principle of parent participation in their children's education is given force of law.

In the United Kingdom the Warnock Committee's Report **Special Educational Needs** (1978) states:

The support, (for parents) . . . must be seen as taking place within a partnership between parents and the members of the different services. To the extent that it enables parents

15

more effectively to help their children at home and at school the support should be an integral part of the provision made for children with special educational needs, which parents have the right to expect. (p. 161)

This Law and this Report recognise that parents wish to have a right to be actively involved in the education of their handicapped children. Moreover, professionals who work with the handicapped increasingly recognise that the family is the primary socialization agent. Research is consistently establishing that parents' child rearing practices, particularly as they relate to language, cognition, motor skills and behaviour control, play quite a vital role in influencing their children's development (Strom, 1974a, 1974b and 1976). Bricker and Bricker (1974) indicate how a parent training programme for both non-delayed and retarded children can help parents by providing them with counselling, with instruction in self-help skills, toileting procedures, language training, motor development, principles of child development, and methods for elimination of undesirable behaviour. By establishing a parent based intervention programme it would appear that effective co-ordination of school programmes, of social work and speech therapy services and programmes of instruction in the home can be achieved. Moreover, Karlsruher (1974) has stressed that a shortage of professionals has now resulted in the recognition that non-professionals can be used most effectively. Once parents become aware of the effects of intervention programmes, then they are likely to develop renewed energy and, along with professionals working in the field, seek to establish ongoing intervention programmes (Abramson et al., 1977; Jeffree & McConkey, 1976a). For example, Allen's maxim that intervention programmes should seek to maximise a child's position within his own growth curve (Allen, 1959) has led to both greater realism by parents and to their increased determination to provide their children with the optimum conditions for development (Karnes, 1969; Kirk, 1958), certainly during their formative years (Sandow and Clarke, 1978; Torrance, 1971). Furthermore, Skeels has emphasised that

Even under present day conditions there are still countless numbers of infants born with sound biological constitutions and with potentialities for development well within the normal range who will become mentally retarded and a burden to society unless appropriate intervention occurs (Skeels, 1966; Skeels and Dye, 1939).

Current findings (e.g. Special Educational Needs, 1978) and past history demonstrate the relevance of intervention and of including parents in multi-disciplinary teams.

PARENTS' NEEDS AND DIFFICULTIES

Teaching and working with parents of intellectually handicapped children involves acquiring an understanding of their distinct needs, their problems and their aspirations, as well as recognising the skills they possess for maximising their children's development. To ignore this highly personal factor especially in long term intervention will most likely reduce or curtail the commitment parents have to such an intervention programme. This personal factor distinguishes the long term, parent-based programmes from those with short-term, limited objectives (see Tables 2.1 and 2.2.).

Karnes and Zehrbach (1972) have indicated that parents of handicapped children recognise the importance of their participation in intervention programmes. Furthermore, they stress that parents benefit personally from these activities and their continued involvement further extends the skills of the professionals. However, involvement of parents of the intellectually handicapped is only likely to be successful if, at the beginning, some of the problems of these parents are closely examined (Murray, 1959). Essentially, as Baker (1977) and Brutten, Richardson and Mangel (1973) have indicated, these basic problems begin with reactions to the birth of a retarded child into a family.

An appreciation of these reactions is necessary for professionals involved in a long term parent intervention programme. Reactions to the birth of an handicapped child are individual. Situations which may present an acute problem to one family may scarcely be noticed in another.

Yet there are general conclusions that can be drawn, such as the different stages of reaction to crises that all families of intellectually handicapped children are thought to experience at one time or another. Professional sensitivity to these reactions is likely to be a key variable — determining to some extent, parents' participation in and perseverance with intervention. However, it should also be stressed that for some parents the crisis of having an exceptional child is one which parents can and do work through without professional help (Matheny and Vernick, 1969). It is Matheny and Vernick's contention that a learning process involving an emotional reorganisation has already been embarked upon by the parents from the instant they become aware, or are told, that their child is different. An understanding by professionals of this learning process and its stages would seem to be imperative in order to maximise parent and professional co-operation.

PARENTS' REACTIONS TO CRISES

Molony (1971) and Shontz (1965) have referred to the different stages of reaction to crises. For example, people experience "shock, realization, defensive retreat and then acknowledgment". Therefore, whenever any parent or group of parents present themselves it is reasonable to expect that they may well be experiencing different stages of this crisis reaction. Professionals running an intervention programme must take account of the possibility of stress resulting from this crisis reaction. However, Heisler (1972) has stated that parents of handicapped children should in no way be regarded as being emotionally disturbed because of the crises they have to live through. It needs to be emphasised that they also experience joy, satisfaction and success and as such seek to live satisfying and productive lives. Parents of handicapped children confront those internal events of anxiety, shock, disappointment, fear, joy and hope, and in so many ways their aspirations for their intellectually handicapped children are similar to their aspirations for their non-handicapped children. Above all, they want to do what they think is right for their intellectually handicapped children. They would like to see themselves as good parents, and they would certainly like others to view them in this light. Professionals need therefore to hold or indeed express a constructive view of the parenting skills of these families with intellectually handicapped children. Similarly, professionals need to be aware of the optimism and apsirations that parents of even the most severely handicapped child have. For example, Baker (1977) writes of her Down's Syndrome baby

... eventually she'll require open heart surgery. If this hurdle is passed we can focus more closely on the mental retardation and help her achieve many goals. ... I no longer feel overcome by the uncertainty of the future ... having a special child isn't so bad. (p. 69-70)

Similar examples and classifications of parental reaction and parental aspiration have been made by Gorham (1975), Haley (1971), Kanner (1952), Losen and Diament (1978) and Michaels and Schuman (1962).

WHEN SHOULD PARENTS BECOME INVOLVED IN AN INTERVENTION PROGRAMME?

Parents of the intellectually handicapped may wish to become involved as soon as the child is born or, if the handicap is caused by accident, as soon as the accident occurs. Simmons-Martin (1976) points out that a parent can feel deep grief when the child is found to be defective and, in some instances, may need to experience a period of mourning. If the intervention programme commences soon after the child's birth then professionals ought to be aware that this "period of mourning" may be in train.

However, in any intervention programme the optimal stage for parents to become involved would appear to be what Molony describes as the "stage of reintegration followed by mature adaptation" (Molony, 1971, p.915). The important part to stress here is that this stage of adaptation and adjustment may well follow stages of depression and denial of the birth or accident. However, **some** parents, despite much emotional stress, can receive quite pessimistic information about their children and then, almost immediately act positively — demonstrating behaviour associated with "mature adaptation". Therefore, it appears that after varied periods of time parents reach a mature acknowledgement and acceptance of the facts of their child's retardation. Then they learn to live with it, to become constructive in planning, and to tolerate it without undue stress (Molony, 1971; Murray 1959). It is clear that it is at this stage of acceptance that parents are most ready to participate in and persevere with a continuing intervention programme. Some parents clearly come to this stage spontaneously, others reach it with help and support. Certainly, any intervention programme must seek to provide that support. It must also be accepted by the professionals involved that many parents **never** achieve this final stage of mature adaptation and intervention programmes may not succeed for this reason. The very opposite of this sense of integration and purpose is clearly a sense of hopelessness. For example, studies such as those of Downey (1965) and Jaslow and Stehman (1966) point out that parents felt that their efforts at caring and teaching were of little purpose as far as improvement in their children's performance was concerned. This feeling of hopelessness can be associated with such characteristic behaviours as parents' loss of self-esteem, much disappointment and ignoring or denying opinions. These factors may affect parents' abilities to teach their children skills. Clearly, any multi-disciplinary team involved in an intervention programme has to listen to and accept these feelings and points of view and not become too discouraged by them or become impatient with parents who manifest them (Murray, 1959; Webster, 1976).

HOW PARENTS ARE TOLD ABOUT THEIR CHILD'S HANDICAP

It appears that the manner in which parents are initially told about their child's handicap is also most important for later adjustment. Parents have drawn attention to the unsatisfactory nature of the manner in which they were told of their child's handicap, and this insensitivity has had lasting results (Baker, 1977; Gayton and Walker, 1974; Johns, 1971; Special Educational Needs, 1978). It is clear that some doctors still present the diagnosis of intellectual handicap as a hopeless one and this attitude lingers on (Golden and Davis, 1974). Furthermore, as Chazan and Laing (1978) indicate, even allowing for the fact that telling parents that their child is handicapped is an extremely difficult and delicate task, many parents surveyed were dissatisfied with the insensitive way in which their child's disability had been revealed to them. Apart from the unnecessary suffering caused, a side effect of clumsy or insensitive disclosure may be embittered relationships between parents, medical and other professional staff, on whose assistance parents will certainly depend in the years ahead. This insensitive disclosure could have long lasting results and thus affect the nature of intervention. Another outcome of this insensitivity and lack of guidance from professionals is that parents may look for less reliable help outside the education, health and welfare services or participate in that process of regular referral to different professionals or agencies (Victorian Committee on Mental Retardation, 1977).

ACCEPTANCE OR ADJUSTMENT TO A CHILD'S HANDICAP?

Buscaglia (1975), Raymond, Slaby and Lieb (1975) and Wing (1972) considered it unrealistic to expect parents to accept children's handicap, if to accept means to feel agreeable about it. Furthermore, Stone (1973) writes that acceptance of the child is not necessarily the goal, for rejection may be the only successful means by which a particular family can adjust. Tymchuk (1975) presents a model for working with parents of the developmentally disabled which combines dynamic and behavioural therapeutic strategies. With the dynamic strategy, there is little systematic effort made to directly involve the parents in the training of their children. Tymchuk implies that the reconciliation of the parents' feelings will somehow translate into their

18

acceptance of their child's behaviour. It is not acceptance that is needed but rather that parents can be helped to both acknowledge the nature and degree of the intellectual handicap and cope with it by aiming for defined attainable goals. An active, continuing supportive role by professionals clearly helps a family's adjustment to the presence of a handicapped child, and best prepares them for achieving attainable goals (Stone 1973). Understanding the nature of this professional supportive role appears imperative in successful intervention and in the provision of continuing education, health and welfare services.

PARENTAL CONCERNS AND ASPIRATIONS: TOWARDS A MODEL OF NORMALITY

Parents of intellectually handicapped children share a range of concerns similar to those parents whose children are developing normally. These parents are concerned about their children's language and social development and about their children's ability to function with increasing independence (McCormack, 1978). Parents of the intellectually handicapped express concern about how their children's language development will affect their social interaction, their overall education and their potential for some measure of future independence. Hunter and Shucman (1967) and Marcus (1977) have written about the coping patterns and styles of adaptation by families with retarded and psychotic children. Similarly, Bice (1952), Green and Soutter (1977) and Parks (1977) recognise the distinct concerns of mothers with intellectually handicapped and cerebral palsied children and make recommendations related to their management and long term care. Other writers in turn make reference to parental aspirations towards models of normality no matter how handicapped the child (Grunewald, 1969; Ray, 1974; Wolfensberger, 1977).

Parental involvement in intervention programmes, in both the short and long term, is initiated and sustained by the **hope** that is engendered when these programmes commence. Galloway and Galloway (1971) refer to the fact that a parent's attendance at introductory intervention programme meetings by no means commits him or her to future attendance. In the vital early sessions there is a clear need to be as realistic as possible about specific goals whilst at the same time dispelling ideas that intellectually handicapped children are permanently limited in their language and social development.

IMPLEMENTING AN INTERVENTION PROGRAMME: COST FACTORS

The development of any intervention programme must depend as much on the economic realisation of objectives as well as on the technical demonstration of the effectiveness of the intervention programme. Home based programmes are generally low cost and therefore have this advantage. Furthermore, there is a definite realisation that intellectually handicapped children reared by their parents demonstrate higher developmental levels compared with intellectually handicapped children reared in institutions (Carr, 1975; Centerwall and Centerwall, 1960; Goldfarb 1943; Lyle, 1960a; Spitz, 1945 and 1946). Melyn and White (1973) showed that variability in the acquisition of language between home reared and institutionally reared Down's Syndrome children was greater than for all other areas of development. Increasingly, therefore, language intervention programmes are likely to be home based and as such could be regarded as cost effective.

WHICH PROFESSIONALS SHOULD BE INVOLVED?

As research in methods of shaping and enhancing the language development of the intellectually handicapped and language delayed child has grown so reports have appeared demonstrating that these teaching techniques can in fact be used by para professionals,

19

particularly parents (Fredericks *et al* 1971; Freeman and Thompson, 1973). Few can dispute that of all the skills the retarded child most needs, the ability to communicate with a reasonable degree of effectiveness is foremost in the achievement of optimum social adjustment.

Schneider and Vallon (1954 and 1955) demonstrated the effectiveness of a school based speech therapy programme for mentally retarded children which can readily be adopted by para professionals. However, they give few details of the therapy programme or of the particular progress made by the children. However, Wood (1964) illustrates how speech therapy activities related to object naming, vocabulary building, articulation and sentence formulation can, in fact, take place in the home.

Social workers had long been involved with families with intellectually handicapped children, providing support services (Goldberg and Neil, 1972; Hewett, 1970; Schild, 1971). Bayley (1973) demonstrates how care by social workers can only be effective when they link in with, and are supported by, the informal caring that goes on throughout society. This linking role is seen to be a distinct contribution by the social workers. For example, Bayley (1973) demonstrates how the social networks of families of the intellectually handicapped were naturally affected by the needs of their intellectually handicapped children. Rees (1978) writes how a combination of service and casework-type activities involve social workers in obtaining day care for mentally handicapped children in nurseries and occupational centres. Webster (1976) emphasises the importance for counsellors in understanding and appreciating the private world of parents with handicapped children, and of being aware of their desire for growth. Rose (1974a and 1974b) writes quite specifically about the role of social workers in devising treatment programmes for the intellectually handicapped in which parents are taught such procedures as positive reinforcement and shaping, extinction, time-out from reinforcement, cueing, modelling and behavioural rehearsal. Furthermore, Rose stresses that when a programme such as this is organised by social workers on a small group basis the cost in staff time per changed behaviour remained "substantially less" than individual or family treatment. However, this view of the importance of work with parents in groups contrasts with the findings of Mira (1970) who emphasises the importance of individual behaviour modification training for both parents and teachers.

Speech therapists, social workers and counsellors are all able to demonstrate and justify their role in providing services for the intellectually handicapped. Furthermore, the training of parents individually or in groups and the provision of parent training manuals are also advocated as effective means of home based intervention (Heifetz, 1977).

BEHAVIOURALLY ORIENTED INTERVENTION PROGRAMMES AND MANUALS

Clearly, studies aimed at involving parents in the treatment of their children have mushroomed in recent years. The most common, or the most publicised, approach has been the application of behaviour modification principles to childhood disorders; and this approach has been described in many articles and reviews (Berkowitz and Graziano, 1973; Hall and Broden, 1967; Hall *et al.* 1972; Johnson and Katz, 1973; O'Dell, 1974; Tramontana, 1971; Ullman and Kemp, 1974; Wahler *et al.* 1969; Zeilberger *et al* 1968). These writings conclude that parents can be trained to effectively modify their children's behavioural disorders. However, few of them examine the effects of intervention beyond a few weeks or months. Fewer still examine the generalisation of behaviour in different stimulus settings. For example, Wahler's (1969) data indicate that parent training with subsequent changes in the children's behaviour at home did not change the children's behaviour in the new stimulus setting at school. Furthermore, Herbert *et al.* (1973) and Sajwaj (1973) emphasise the difficulties in the use of behavioural techniques by parents and the failures that can result.

Despite the reservations of these writers and, presumably, the many unreported projects which have failed, as well as the tendency of journals to reject papers dealing with negative results (Greenwald, 1975; Walster and Cleary, 1970), there has been an outpouring of parental guides and manuals (Becker, 1971; Hall, 1971; McIntyre, 1970; Patterson, 1971; Patterson and Gullion, 1971; Vallett, 1969; Watson, 1974; Williams and Jaffa, 1971). Moreover, other manuals and guides have been produced which, while not explicitly under the title of behaviour modification programmes, do make detailed reference to the terminology and techniques of behaviour modification (e.g. Cunningham and Sloper, 1978; Hare and Hare, 1977; Heisler, 1972; Webster, 1977). It appears therefore that the production of a parent training manual is essential. For example, Heifetz (1977) has indicated that for a home based intervention programme manuals and group meetings provide continuity between programme stages and may be an optimum method of training. Specific training programmes for parent groups have also been produced (e.g. Benassi and Benassi, 1973; Cunningham and Jeffree, 1975; Eyeberg and Johnson, 1974; Galloway and Galloway, 1971; Mash et al. 1973; Patterson, Cobb and Rar, 1973; Peine and Munro, 1973). Similarly, multi-media presentations and programmed packages such as Karlins (1972); Latham and Hofmeister (1973); Shearer and Shearer (1972); White and Haring (1976) are now readily available. However, few of these manuals and multi-media packages have been carefully evaluated by parents or other prospective users. Rather the scene is one of competing claims being made by different authors. For parents, some confusion naturally ensues.

USING PROGRAMME MATERIALS EFFECTIVELY

If parents of the intellectually handicapped are to use these materials effectively, there is a definite need for the programmes to be explicit about defining critical training variables such as (i) the role of group discussions, (ii) the role of lectures, (iii) the role of modelling techniques, (iv) the role of reading assignments. These variables are referred to but their particular function is not carefully described. There is also a need for explicit description of training techniques and programme contents in relation to both parent variables and different etiologies of intellectual handicap. Above all, parents need quite definite advice about the extent to which skills taught do, in fact, generalise to other stimulus settings and also that the teaching programmes may well need to be maintained over many years, if not over a lifetime. Except for Cunningham and Sloper's "Helping Your Handicapped Baby" (Cunningham and Sloper, 1978) little reference is made to generalisation of skills and long term maintenance of a programme by those writers who advocate intervention to develop the language and social skills of the intellectually handicapped.

Parents need to know that the strategies of behaviour modification are well suited to precise short term behavioural objectives in which immediate environmental contingencies can be taken into account (Keller and Ribes-Inesta, 1974). As such, behaviour modification offers a rationale for the treatment of many behavioural disorders. Yet for parents of the intellectually handicapped, its applicability may well be limited because these parents must be concerned with long term objectives and sustained treatment. They do not have the solace that after the treatment the child will be normal. Manuals make no reference to this factor. Therefore, essential issues for training parents of intellectually handicapped children are factors such as generalisation, long-term maintenance of training and close examination of training-method and parent attitudes (see Table 2.3).

What should be the goals of a parent training programme? What should be the language teaching goals for the children once their parents have mastered particular teaching techniques? These are questions that parents want answered and that they feel can best be answered if they are involved in an intervention programme from the outset. Murray (1959) has stressed that parents do feel the need to do something themselves for their child. Therefore, by involving parents, by teaching them the principles of structured teaching and behaviour modification, and by encouraging them to apply these with their children, it is likely that the parent teaching system developed will be both adaptable and more easily maintained. Furthermore, these factors are integral to the procedural control that Zifferblatt regards as necessary for the teaching of a skill (Zifferblatt, 1973). The manuals do not indicate how this procedural control can be achieved.

In a home based setting, there is a need to supply outline manuals of tasks to be taught. It is necessary to ensure that the language of the manuals is jargon free and understood by parents; and to provide parents with clear information about the variety and relationships of professional support services. Parental confusion about these different services can so easily lead to lowering of morale and reduction in the level of participation and therefore a failure to establish procedural control.

DISTINCTIVE CHARACTERISTICS OF THE GOALS, CONTENT AND FUNCTION OF A LANGUAGE INTERVENTION TRAINING PROGRAMME

The goals and content of service based language programmes for the intellectually handicapped are many and varied. They must take account of particular teaching preferences, of the role of the children's physical and cognitive development, and of research evidence of factors which determine the language development of the severely handicapped. Home based teaching programmes necessarily include such issues as (a) contracts with families, (b) the role of weekly group meetings, and of weekly individual family sessions with therapist-consultants, (c) the role of language assessment procedures for both parents and therapists, (d) the use of videotapes in clinic and home, (e) parental reports of their children's behaviour, (f) the development of skills by parents in observing, recording, targeting and tracking behaviour, and (g) the completing of various exercises, such as devising simple teaching programmes for achieving specific target behaviours (Berkowitz and Graziano, 1973; Cartwright, 1968; Patterson and Gullion, 1971; Rose, 1974a and 1974b).

Parent group training involves role-playing, modelling and discussions on the use of social reinforcement, including token systems and time-out procedures. Yet these factors may be contrary to the usual family domestic routine. However, there is evidence (Cartwright, 1968, and Rose, 1974b) that the small group, when highly attractive to its members, provides considerable pressure on them to conform to therapeutic demands and group norms. In such an instructional setting a small parent group can be a source of extensive ideas for reinforcement and for developing other teaching plans. In addition, multiple membership also permits many different types of co-actors in role-playing which, in itself, is an important training procedure. Parents in groups help to maintain each other's high level of enthusiasm for a programme and they provide abundant social reinforcement for each other's achievements. These factors may determine whether a group not only stays together but whether individual parents are able to sustain their teaching. However even if group training is most economic, there are many occasions when parent withdrawal from the group is necessary. Patterson *et al.* (1973) illustrate how, if the target behaviour that they were trying to eliminate persisted after many weeks, parents were removed from the group and tailor-made procedures were developed and applied on an individual family basis. The authors reported data and statistical analyses of both the reliability of their behavioural measures and the significance of the behavioural changes in the families in both small group and individual settings. The opportunity for parents to withdraw from groups to receive individual tuition may not only determine their success but may also in turn contribute to the success of the group. This factor is not referred to by Rose (1974b) or indeed by other advocates of group training such as Eyeberg and Johnson (1974) or Peine and Munro (1973).

Walder *et al.* (1971) were concerned about **maintaining** parent involvement. The importance of the Walder *et al.* study lies not only in the authors' development and illustration of behaviour modification approaches to family therapy, but also in their co-ordinated, clearly sequenced, teaching process for working with large numbers of families. Above all, they appear to have come close to creating an educational curriculum through which parents can be educated to maintain independent application of principles. The maintenance of parent involvement over many years and the development of controlled teaching procedures which can become part of domestic routine are referred to by very few writers (see Table 2.2). Berkowitz and Graziano (1973) stress that Walder is an investigator " . . . who has carried out controlled comparisons of parents trained in operant approaches with those families treated through more traditional psychodynamics". Walder's comparative study is an application to parents of the effectiveness of behavioural strategies versus other therapies and compares with a smaller comparative study by Lazarus which found in favour of a structured behavioural programme compared with other therapies (Lazarus, 1966).

Despite the attractiveness of external consequences for parent participation in a structured behaviour modification programme which many writers emphasise (Watson, 1969; and Wolpe, 1976), it is necessary to remember how self evaluative and self produced reactions can take precedence over external consequences. Behaviourists such as Rachlin (1976) do remain staunchly opposed to the notion that behaviour, however complex, can be influenced by cognitions. However, any analysis of results from long term parent programmes must take into account, even for simple behavioural change, and certainly in relation to change in parent attitudes, the fact that conditioning is ultimately produced through the operation of higher mental processes by cognitive mediation (Bandura, 1973 and 1974, and Brewer, 1974). A failure to recognise this by professionals and evaluators alike is to demonstrate a lack of awareness of the distinctive characteristics of parental roles. This lack of awareness can easily lead to a programme's demise. Apart from Walder's writing, few references are made to the processes by which changes in parental attitudes and skills occur.

THE LANGUAGE PROBLEMS OF THE INTELLECTUALLY HANDICAPPED

The evidence that intervention programmes, and particularly parent oriented intervention programmes, are likely to benefit the intellectually handicapped, appears overwhelming. Mittler has been quite explicit that we cannot simply sit back and wait for language to develop (Mittler, 1975). Enough is now known to suggest that language does not develop merely by the provision of a stimulating, enriched, environment (Renfrew, 1972).

That the intellectually handicapped in general, and the more severely handicapped in particular, have distinct problems with language, has been recognised for some time. Reviews dealing with the overall problem of definite lags in the language development of the intellectually handicapped have appeared with regularity (e.g. Andrews and Andrews, 1974; Blount, 1968; Goertzen, 1957; Gould, 1976; Harrison, 1958; Karlin and Strazzula, 1952; Spradlin, 1963a and 1963b; Spreen, 1965a and 1965b). Yet, incidence statistics of language dysfunction do not seem to provide adequate support for the interpretation that language development is poor because intelligence is low or, indeed, that language and intelligence are interdependent to such an extent that they may be, to all intents and purposes, regarded as the same process (Spreen, 1965a). Nevertheless, Dentler and Mackler (1962) found a correlation coefficient of 0.48 (with C.A. held constant) between the complete Parson Language Sample (a test which samples various types of communicatory behaviour, including gestural non-vocal behaviour as well as language understanding, comprehension and repetition) and the Porteus Maze Test, which is considered by Dentler and Mackler to be a non-verbal indicator of intelligence.

This result seems to confirm a moderate relationship between language and intelligence and other writers have confirmed this relationship, particularly with the more severely retarded (Clarke and Clarke, 1974). Spreen (1965a) emphasises that onset of talking, speech sound development and acquisition of phonemes show a rather low, but consistently observed, correlation with standard intelligence tests. Relatively high correlations are obtained between intelligence and measurements of vocabulary up to a mental age of seven or eight. This illustrates what Piaget (1926) and Vygotsky (1962) have to say about egocentrism of both language and thought in the young child; namely, that in communication as well as language structure, children seem bound by their development levels.

23

Speech productivity, i.e. measures of the number of words or the number of different words spoken during a particular interaction, shows only a moderate relationship with both intelligence and vocabulary level. Parents in a language based intervention are keen to know this (Kimber and Porritt, 1976). In most of the reports of the relationship between IQ measures and speech productivity (Budoff and Purseglove, 1963; Dunn and Hottell, 1961; Gould, 1976; Ho and White, 1963) a standard IQ measure, the Stanford Binet Form L.M. or the Full Scale W.I.S.C. IQ, is used and it is found that the correlation coefficients tend to decrease when non-verbal measures of intelligence are employed (Gould, 1976; Wing, 1975).

Just as parents raise questions about the relationship between intelligence and language acquisition so they are concerned as to whether there are differences between etiologies of intellectual handicap or indeed between boys and girls. Variables such as these might indicate that a child would fare better or worse in an intervention programme according to whether the subject was a Down's Syndrome boy, a brain damaged girl or familial retarded boy. Lyle's work (Lyle, 1959) highlighted the language differences between Down's and non-Down's Syndrome intellectually handicapped children in institutions, and Gallagher (1957) compared the language performance of brain injured and non-brain injured retarded children. Yet these studies are of institutionalised children and in Karlin and Strazzula's terms, institutionalised children live in a very sheltered, protective and tense environments (Karlin and Strazzula, 1952) and it could be expected that a more open and stimulating environment at home would result in different language attainment. For example, Fried (1977), Johnson and Olley (1971), Schneider and Vallon (1955) make comparisons of the language development of Down's syndrome, non-Down's syndrome and brain damaged subjects and provided they were matched on C.A. and M.A. then no statistically significant difference was found. Conflicting results appear when comparisons of familial mentally handicapped and other mentally handicapped subjects are made. However, these conflicting results may just occur because of different definitions of familial mentally handicapped subjects (Haring and Cohen (1975); Robinson (1976); York and Williams (1977)). When comparable comparisons are made, then superiority in language development favours the familial retards particularly when compared with Down's syndrome children (Johnson and Olley, 1971). Yet these studies make no reference to the influence of motivation on language development, particularly with reference to the language skills of Down's syndrome children, yet Lenneberg (1967) considers this to be a most important variable.

Various writers (Fried, 1977; Schneider and Vallon, 1954; Spreen 1965a) make reference to the fact that no difference in the language development of boys and girls could or should be expected. However, in any case work, the child's sex is identified and the influence of this sex factor in language development is raised by parents (Kimber and Porritt, 1976).

Menyuk (1971), writing about deviant language behaviour, states that the only variables which appear to affect the acquisition of the linguistic system by most children, are age and the complexities of the linguistic system. Lenneberg (1967) and Reynell (1972) are concerned that it is advantageous to intervene early because there is less chance that deviant language behaviour will have become established. For many writers, 18 months of age apppears as a dividing line between less and more complex language. For example, Flavell (1963) states that from 18 months onwards a child starts to make symbolic representations of sensory motor problems. Menyuk (1971) writes that from 18 months onwards a child progresses from babbling and producing single words to producing two to three word phrases. Eisenson (1980) writes that at approximately 18 months of age a child can produce three to fifty single words and that beyond this age the child uses syntactic features similar to those used by adults. By 36 months a child understands most of what is said by a "reasonable adult". However, this developmental information about the increasing complexities of language beyond 18 months of age only implies that intervention may be more difficult with the child at a more advanced stage of language development. It is assumption rather than fact that intervention with children at an early stage of language development is likely to be more successful than with children at a more advanced stage. Parents of older intellectually handicapped children who are functioning above or well above a measured language age of 18 months are concerned as to whether the older child will respond as much to intervention as the young child, who is at a more primitive level of language development.

Advances in language teaching particularly in relationship to the careful subdivision between receptive and expressive language have occurred. However, traditional feelings about the speech development of different groups of intellectually handicapped children die hard. These feelings are shown for example, in the views of Stinchfield and Young (1947) that

mental subnormality is still a fact and when a child fails to learn to talk because of real mental deficiency, hope is still an illusion and must remain so under the limitations of our present knowledge. (p. 47)

Similarly West, Kennedy and Young (1947) stated that

the true mongol is particularly unresponsive to speech rehabilitation and it is practically useless to attempt such training. Rehabilitation of speech of the mongol, therefore should be undertaken only with the clear understanding of everyone concerned that the therapy is experimental and any possible results will be meagre and in proportion to the patient's level of intelligence. (p. 29)

This pessimistic attitude may need to be considered as an important variable in the assessment of performance (Carrow, 1972). For example, Lenneberg (1967) makes the point, particularly in regard to the articulation skills of intellectually handicapped Down's syndrome children, that their indifferent speech development may be due to their poor motivation and the poor expectations of their parents rather than to insurmountable physical difficulties.

RECEPTIVE LANGUAGE AND ITS RELATIONSHIP TO EXPRESSIVE LANGUAGE

Schneider and Vallon (1955) at the conclusion of their speech therapy programme wrote that

one cannot measure the degree of progress in language development of a child who did not speak prior to therapy by the number of words he has learned to say, because various other factors such as the degree to which the child has learned to use them purposefully, the various language concepts that have been established . . . tends to make such an evaluation misleading and invalid. (p. 420)

Since then, reference to receptive language skills has been made both qualitatively and quantitatively. Fried (1977) and the Developmental Language Study of Cooper, Moodley and Reynell (1979) present separate age scores for receptive and expressive language. The division of language skills also appears in case studies, e.g. Berry (1976); Berry and Foxen (1978). This attention in case studies to receptive and expressive language, and in particular to cueing relevant behaviour as something analogous to developing comprehension skills, is exemplified by Salzinger, Feldman and Portnoy (1970) in their training programme for parents of brain damaged children. In particular, attention has also been given to the teaching of comprehension skills by Herriott (1970) and Mittler (1974).

If the language problems of the severely intellectually handicapped are distinctive, what particular language skills should be taught? Above all, what experiences do parents provide for their children that are relevant to their children's level of language and cognitive development? Advocates of language intervention programmes from Schneider and Vallon (1954) to Renfrew (1972) and Cooper and Moodley and Reynell (1978) fail to give specific answers to these questions. A speech therapist's advice "You must keep talking to your child . . . and use lots of stimulating language" may be laudable but it ignores the fact that development of language for the intellectually handicapped is more slow moving and needs to be carefully sequenced. A major criticism of much of the literature is that this characteristic of the language development of the intellectually handicapped is not explicitly recognised except by writers such as Mittler (1975) or Sailor, Guess and Baer (1973).

In terms of just what can be taught, it is clear that the elements of the language system can be taught long before the child actually starts to speak. Mash and Terdal (1973) and Seitz and Riedel (1974) emphasise the role of listening skills and the importance of parent-child interactions as the teaching target. Similarly Mittler (1974) is concerned about teachers and parents having proof that children understand the "language of instruction". In this context, Friedlander (1970) makes a significant point about the difference between listening and speaking. "The speaker has total freedom to control the formulations of his message while the listener must accommodate his listening processing tactics to the requirements of the message." This point is, of course, most pertinent in the teaching of receptive language skills to the intellectually handicapped. Friedlander is talking about the development of speaking and listening in normal people and it is necessary to translate the notion to severely mentally retarded children with severe language problems. However, he is explicit that listening to and establishing understanding of the speech of others is fundamental to the development of spoken language. These listening and comprehension skills can be taught, as MacDonald and his team demonstrate (MacDonald *et al.* 1974). Yet, for these intellectually handicapped children to acquire listening skills and develop comprehension, a teaching programme must pay attention to providing relevant non-linguistic and non-verbal cues (Mittler, 1970). This role of non-linguistic and non-verbal cues in developing children's receptive language skills receives little specific attention by such writers as Miller and Yoder (1972b), Sinclair (1973), and Watson (1974), although this criticism cannot be made of the detailed work of Bricker and Bricker (1974) and Lovaas *et al.* (1966 and 1973), or Schiefelbusch (1963).

STRUCTURE, SEQUENCE AND DEVELOPMENTAL CAPABILITIES IN A LANGUAGE PROGRAMME

Bricker and Bricker (1974) emphasise the key role of structure in any effective language intervention programme. They emphasise that this decision is based on many years of work, during which they have attempted to integrate operant, linguistic, cognitive and psycholinguistic approaches to both language acquisition and language training. They apply these approaches to children whose language is moderately to severely developmentally delayed. The Brickers indicate the importance of the pre-linguistic forms of behaviour for subsequent language acquisition. The early language training strategy is based on the sensorimotor lattice structure which indicates the primary sequential forms of behaviour and the prerequisite behaviours for each task. It appears that these processes, which are not linguistic in a formal sense, and certainly not verbal, constitute the initial basis for the development of functional language. Physiotherapists such as Hughes (1971) demonstrate how the acquisition of physical skills form the basis of a handicapped baby being able to attend. This in turn is the basis for the development of later communication skills.

The developmental literature stresses that language content should be taught in sequence patterned on normal development. Flavell (1971) points out that Piaget has stood firm in this central thesis and that the sequential aspect is inevitable. Considerable research has been undertaken with intellectually handicapped children to see if they follow the same order of cognitive stages at a slowed down rate, and in general, this viewpoint has supported Piaget's position (Kessler, 1970; Piaget, 1954; Piaget and Inhelder, 1971; Woodward 1959). For example, for Piaget (1951) the appearance of the first question forms indicates a significant movement towards the formation of concepts or socialised thought and communication or socialised language. However, it should be stressed that Piaget finds language to be subordinate to thought in that "these superstructures of propositional logic go beyond the language of the subject and cannot even be formulated by means of the current language alone" (Piaget, 1963). Yet, Reynell, whose developmental language scales were used in this research finds language to be 'a true vehicle of thought' (Reynell, 1969b).

Kessler emphasises the need to incorporate a Piagetian view of conceptual development into language training and, as such provides a supporting theoretical basis for beginning a language programme with sensorimotor tasks. This point of view is also supported by Snyder and McLean (1976) in their analysis of deficient language acquisition strategies by E.M.R. children. A problem in understanding children's language acquisition strategies is whether these sensorimotor tasks in turn lead to conceptual thinking and functional language usage.

Writings by Bloom (1970); Brown (1973); Sailor, Guess and Baer (1973) and Slobin (1973) provide evidence that both content and developmental progressions in language programmes for intellectually handicapped children are similar to those seen in models of normal development. However, these writers do not provide strong empirical evidence of the links between sensorimotor tasks, the onset of receptive language understanding, and above all, the links between comprehension and the production of one and two word utterances and ultimately simple sentences.

Of relevance here is a controversy concerning the cognitive functioning of mentally retarded individuals as compared to non retarded individuals. One group, the developmental theorists such as Zigler (1969), maintain that individuals differing in rate of intellectual development as measured by IQ but equal in level of development as measured by MA will not differ in cognitive skills that are inherently related to IQ. The opposing group, the difference theorists such as Milgram (1973) contended that the mentally retarded will manifest inferior cognitive performance when compared to non-retarded individuals of the same MA. Any differences in test performance between EMR subjects and non-retarded subjects could be interpreted as support for the difference theoretical position. However, the proven performance of the EMR group could be attributed to an experiential deficit and any differences in test performances should not be construed as a genuine cognitive difference if the two groups differ markedly in test-related experience. This is of relevance in any comparison of the effects on children's language development of difference teaching programmes.

THE NATURE OF LANGUAGE TEACHING

The language building programmes of Lovaas et al. (1966), with their defined range of language forms: labels, mands, verbs, pronouns and prepositions, demonstrated the ever widening range of language teaching. Identifying these language forms would appear to be imperative. Yet, once this has been done, if a programme then places its emphasis on understanding, on the development of receptive language, will this form the basis for the development of expressive language, of speech? Guess and Baer have in part demonstrated a functional independence of these two modalities (Guess and Baer, 1973; Rees, 1978). However, because parents naturally measure the success of a language teaching programme on whether a child learns to talk, it is imperative to demonstrate the relationship between receptive and expressive language. Once this has been done then concentrating on teaching receptive language skills is more acceptable. Again few programmes, and not even the much used Portage Project (Shearer and Shearer, 1972), are explicit about this relationship or indeed demonstrate just what constitutes receptive language skills.

In the content of any programme, account should be taken of the relationships between sensorimotor tasks, the development of receptive language understanding and, ultimately, of situation relevant speech. Various experimental testings over a number of years need to take place before claims can be made: (i) that low order motor tasks should form the starting point of a language intervention programme; (ii) that these low order motor tasks form the basis for later conceptual and expressive language development; (iii) that the relationship between the acquisition of the linguistic system, the grammar of the language, and the children's physiological and psychological capabilities is understood, and (iv) that there is a stage at which particular language skills generalise. For example, teaching a child to acquire two-word open-pivot utterances (Jeffree et al. 1972) in a clinic oriented teaching situation may be fine, but will this skill generalise and be maintained? Unfortunately most published language teaching programmes (see Table 2.2) are of such limited duration that only very selected aspects of these comprehensive questions can be answered.

A further important question related to both content and method of teaching is whether language development for a heterogeneous sample of intellectually handicapped children is a process of gradual but continuous qualitative and quantitative change, or whether it is in fact characterised by abrupt, uneven, discontinuous changes which are qualitatively different from one another? Certainly, this is a question which parents want answered, and the question is central to the defining of language tasks for a comprehensive programme. Answers to this question may develop greater understanding, and, as such, more sensitive teaching programmes may result. Gray and Ryan (1973) argue that language programmes do not have specific sequential order. It does seem, however, that goals of terminal behaviour must be quite specific within each programme phase and that this notion of limited prescribed goals is what really matters in an effective language programme. It is evident that these limited terminal behaviours (whether they be a sensorimotor grasping skill, matching skill, single word or verb-noun utterance) can be taught (Bidder, Bryant and Gray, 1975; Jacobson, Bernal and Lopes, 1973; Latham and Hofmeister, 1973).

Criticism is made that these goals are so limited that they are unreal, but it is argued that the acquisition of these goals is better than no acquisition at all. Furthermore, for each intellectually handicapped individual, it ought to be possible to determine empirically which particular goals are likely to facilitate language acquisition within the parameters of a developmental language model, no matter whether the model represents a gradual or uneven process. Detailed single case studies similar to that undertaken by Butterfield and Parsons (1973) in regard to the development of chewing skills; or Berry, Mathams and Middleton's study (1977) of a mother and child developing communication skills; or factor analysis of the distinct language abilities of the intellectually handicapped similar to that undertaken by Evans (1977) do provide some answers to the distinct process of language acquisition by the intellectually handicapped. However, these studies concentrate more on the product deficits associated with retarded children's language development and only make passing reference to the deficient acquisition strategies.

What is apparent is that if the item-by-item language increments or terminal goals are crude then children will get fixed on specific tasks and across a sample of intellectually handicapped children language development will be consistent, but developmentally uneven. The more sensitive and refined the language increments the more variability across the sample will be the rule, and language development will be less abrupt. Steady and constant language acquisition and development would appear to depend on language tasks that are limited, sensitive and refined.

DIFFERENT APPROACHES TO TEACHING SPEECH AND LANGUAGE

Effective language intervention can take several forms. One method is to observe the language production of the intellectually handicapped child and to analyse this so that the language teacher or speech therapist can determine and apply those types of inputs which might facilitate the acquisition of more complex language. This might be called a "child centred" developmental approach (Bowerman 1974; Cooper et al., 1974 and 1978; Slobin 1973). Another approach closely allied to this is to make use of imaginative and representational play along with appropriate stimulation within living environments (Jeffree and McConkey, 1974; Strain, 1975). A third approach is essentially concerned with behaviour modification. This provides techniques for specifically organising clinical teaching sessions so that the appropriate language behaviours occur and are strengthened (Bendebba, 1973; Edlund, 1971).

(i) The Role of Development and Cognition

The "child centred" approach epitomized by the writings of Cooper et al. (1974 and 1978), Karlin and Strazzulla (1952) and Wood (1954 and 1964) allows the child to give the lead and then relies on the language teacher or speech therapist to stimulate, correct, or modify the communication skills that children produce. This particular approach represents hypotheses about children's innate intellectual abilities that determine how and when they acquire language. As such, it represents hypotheses that the child's (innate) behaviour helps determine both the content and pace of the language programme (Menyuk, 1971). Here there is a definite emphasis on the role of cognitive development in the acquisition of language similar to that demonstrated by Sinclair (1973). For example, the assumption is that the semantic relations between words that are coded in children's messages reflect underlying conceptual relationships. It is clear that children do not learn the relations between objects through language because children show that they already know something about the ways objects relate to each other long before they use linguistic forms to code such relations (Bloom, 1973). This position emphasises that children need to have formed relational concepts as a necessary (and not simply sufficient) condition for learning the linguistic forms (words and multi-word structures) that encode such concepts. However, this relationship between conceptual development and language development is given little emphasis by those such as Cooper, Moodley and Reynell (1974) and it is not an issue which is examined in the manuals which claim to be able to teach language and social skills (Ullman and Kemp, 1974; White and Haring, 1976).

Staats (1971) has pointed out that this notion of teaching concepts does not recognise the parent's role in developing children's conceptual skills. Certainly it has received much less emphasis than the notion that parents ought to, or could, be a child's primary trainer. The approach which emphasises the importance of teaching concepts relies on the teacher/therapist being able to identify those behaviours which help the child, if necessary, to move through stages of visual control, physical control, to linguistic control over his environment. These pre-linguistic and linguistic behaviours are seen to be facilitated by parents, teachers and other children in the environment. It is an approach to teaching which stresses that young children are exploring their environment and synthesising a sensorimotor and conceptual account of it. However, this approach pre-supposes that parents have a knowledge of child development, have developed skills of observation and assessment, and furthermore, that parents recognise the likely effect on development of their child's handicap (Andrews and Andrews, 1974). However, many other advocates of developmental and cognitive models of speech therapy assume pre-existing skills rather than advocate their teaching as critical for the success of the intervention.

The child centred developmental programme does allow for a system of graded intervention techniques based on normal developmental models (Wood, 1964). It is an approach to language teaching which relies on the Piagetian notion that cognitive structure can be used to explain language acquisition (Karlin and Strazzulla, 1952; Reynell 1969a; Reynell 1972). It is an approach which assumes that the ideal training programme must be capable of adjusting to a given subject's level of cognitive functioning. The assumption is that whatever is taught by a speech therapist is, at any language level, a function of the intellectually handicapped child's cognitive structure. A major obstacle here would appear to be the assessment of a child's cognitive ability prior to and during training. No reference to this difficulty is made by those who are advocates of this method of speech therapy (Jeffree and McConkey, 1974; Wood, 1964).

What are the cognitive prerequisites necessary for intellectually handicapped children to acquire and maintain functional use of speech? Consideration of this question implies that specific cognitive functions or behaviours control a range of linguistic behaviours. As such, this teaching approach (Cooper et al., 1974 and 1978; Weikart et al., 1970 and 1974) assigns primary emphasis to the cognitive system which, in turn, is considered to determine language development. Again, assumptions are made about cognitive prerequisites. References are made to them and yet exactly what is distinctive about the cognitive system of the intellectually handicapped is not spelt out.

(ii) The Role of Play
A second intervention strategy closely allied to the cognitive model is the use that is made of imaginative and representational play. While there is no generally accepted or acceptable definition of play, Jeffree and McConkey (1974), Miller and Yoder (1972a and 1972b) and Morehead (1972) emphasise the importance of the role of play. They all point out that play

within stimulating environments forms an important foundation for cognitive and linguistic development. Tizard *et al.*, (1976a and 1976b) describe the effects of play on child language and social development. They describe the effects of chronological age, of sex, IQ, and social class on children's play and subsequent language development. They identify play as the most obvious body of spontaneous cognitive behaviour from which to draw their conclusions. They found that only two-thirds of free play is spent in playing — the rest is spent observing or listening. The majority of the children's games were brief and, what is most important, their games were accompanied by **talk** to other children. Naturally parents find the notion of play as a basis for language development to be most acceptable. Yet the play of the intellectually handicapped is stereotyped; they don't possess the listening skills referred to by Tizard *et al.* (1976a and 1976b) and they do not spontaneously observe as has been demonstrated by Strain, (1975).

The "child centred" approach of the cognitive theorists, of certain speech therapists, and of those who stress the importance of play in the development of language, are approaches which say little about any systematic method for analysing children's language production. Moreover, there are few guidelines for determining the detailed and sensitive types of inputs that might facilitate the acquisition of more complex language. These approaches appear to say little about shaping a child's behaviour and they presume a somewhat passive role by the teacher, speech therapist or parent.

(iii) The Role of Operant Conditioning

The third language teaching method that has been used is essentially an operant one. Operants are behaviours that can be strengthened by their consequences. For example, the frequency of relevant speech can be increased or decreased by the environment. Sailor, Guess and Baer (1973) employ a comprehensive model using operant conditioning procedures for training language skills in speech deficient children. Bettison (1973) and Brown (1972) demonstrate and recommend similar procedures and Irvine (1976) stresses the need for a data based approach to diagnosis and teaching. The use of operant techniques and the operant nature of language had already been affirmed by Skinner (1957). Salzinger *et al.*, (1962) demonstrated how children's language could be regarded as a reinforceable behaviour. Risley and Wolf (1967) demonstrated how to shape echoic verbalisations into meaningful words. Since then, Schumaker and Sherman (1970) have examined the grammatical structures which could generalise to untrained instances in the case of rules of pluralisation and of past and present verb tenses. Wheeler and Sulzer (1970) taught a generalised skill of complete sentence constructions in place of the "telegraphic" speech by a child. Sailor and Taman (1972) developed stimulus control procedures to establish the relational skills implicit in the accurate use of prepositions. Following these studies, Bidder, Bryant and Gray (1975) demonstrated that the speech of Down's syndrome children could be improved by teaching their mothers how to effectively use positive reinforcement. Concurrent with all these developments, Staats (1968) presented a thorough and detailed revision of experimental language targets, even in complex tasks. Staats' (1968) findings from experimental language studies, and his emphasis on structure and identifying language targets, have quite direct applicability for developing home based behaviour modification programmes. Yet these programmes are often of quite short duration, sometimes lasting for only a few weeks (see Table 2.2). They are task specific and are not sequential in the sense that the mastery of one task will form the basis for the acquisition of the following task. The behaviour modification programmes are often single subject case studies in which no reference is made to the maintenance and generalisation of language skills and, except for a few examples (e.g. Cooper, Moodley and Reynell 1979 or Lovaas, Koegel, Simmons and Long 1973) there is little evidence of follow up.

OPPOSITION TO BEHAVIOUR MODIFICATION PROGRAMMES

It has been mentioned above that many behaviour modification programmes that fail are probably not published, and certainly little reference is made to the reasons for opposition to the use of behaviour modification techniques (Tharp and Wetzel, 1970). Among the opposition issues that need to be examined in a home based programme are (i) why parents might view systematic desensitisation or behaviour modification as unnatural; (ii) why they might regard positive reinforcement as bribery; (iii) why parents have a preference for aversive control — "That child does what he does because I tell him to!" and (iv) why household routines are obstacles to the development and practice of daily monitoring of children's behaviour.

It is clear that parents can only be asked to behave in ways which are compatible with their roles. Salzinger *et al.*, (1970) have written about the limitations in the use of parents as therapists. Hawkins *et al.*, (1966) have emphasised that one of the limitations of parental involvement is the requirement of co-operative parents. However, changing parental roles and styles of interaction with their children, can be achieved in small steps. In contrast, Gajzago and Prior (1974) emphasise the importance of near total change in parenting behaviour in order to remediate the deviant behaviour in particular cases. However, it is evident that for most parents goals must be limited, and roles and lifestyles can and should be changed gradually. This is largely because motivation to continue with change is dependent on success. The attraction of a carefully structured programme is that success on limited behaviour modification tasks can be guaranteed, or that if a particular programme is unsuccessful, the cause is a defect in the programme and not in the child. However, this success is so often **hard won** and parents want the teaching to continue over many months and years, if not the school life of their children.

THE EFFECTIVENESS OF INTERVENTIONS

Table 2.1 identifies a range of studies undertaken during the 1970's to survey and facilitate the language and social skills of the intellectually handicapped. Table 2.2 describes these studies according to their general aims, the length of time the teacher or researchers were involved, the number and age of the children involved. This table has been prepared because titles of papers can sometimes be misleading or because summaries often do not give details of age and etiology of subjects or the length of time parents and therapists are involved. Parents want to know what the nature of their commitment will be and whether evidence exists that the teaching advocated and the goals set can be achieved for children of similar age, sex and etiology.

Seventy studies are examined in Tables 2.1 and 2.2. Some that purport to be descriptions of families coping with the problems of rearing intellectually handicapped children turn out to be surveys of parents' needs and difficulties or the identification of particular children's language skills or difficulties e.g. Abramson, Grovink, Abramson and Sommers (1977), Berry (1976), Prior (1977) Skelton (1972), Sommers and Starkey (1977) and Stone (1973). Others that purport to provide interventions turn out to be general descriptions of services and identification of factors that might determine their success e.g. Gayton and Walker (1974); Golden, Hermine and Pashayan (1976); Sosne, Handleman and Harris (1979); Stone and Chesney (1978); Tein (1977); and Urban (1978). Forty-eight of these studies are concerned with specific interventions. Of these thirty (62 per cent) are concerned with providing behaviour modification programmes, six (13 per cent) with a cognitive developmental programmes, six (12 per cent) with the role of play and 6 (12 per cent) with stressing the role of home visits by social workers and counsellors. While this may not be regarded as a representative sample, it does reflect the dominance of behaviour modification programmes. However, in these 30 behaviour modification programmes, the average period of intervention is for only 2½ months with a range from one week for one subject to 24 weeks for 16 subjects. Each of these behaviour modification programmes demonstrates the success of the interventions. They are programmes in which families and therapists have used selective reinforcement to increase the productive behaviour of the children. They have in turn demonstrated the principle that motivation is determined by contingencies of reinforcement. However, their objectives have been very specific, the time period has been quite limited and apparently none of the interventions failed. Parents of the intellectually handicapped are naturally sceptical about this, even though in theory they do accept that in a suitably arranged environment desired effects can occur without fail. There may be criticism of the developmentally oriented five year study of Cooper, Moodley and Reynell

31

TABLE 2.1

CODE FOR INTERVENTION AND SURVEY STUDIES REVIEWED

Author/Authors, Date	Code
Abramson, Grovink, Abramson and Sommers (1977)	(A,G,A, & S 77)
Benassi and Benassi (1973)	(B & B 73)
Bendebba (1973)	(Ben 73)
Berry (1976)	(B 76)
Berry, Mathams and Middleton (1977)	(B,M & M 77)
Bettison (1974)	(Be 74)
Beveridge, Spencer and Mittler (1978)	(B,S & M 78)
Bidder, Bryant and Gray (1975)	(Bi, Br, & G 75)
Butterfield and Parson (1973)	(Bu & P 73)
Clunies-Ross (1976)	(Cl.R 76)
Cooper, Moodley and Reynell (1974)	(C, M & R 74)
Cooper, Moodley and Reynell (1979)	(C, M & R 79)
Cromer (1972)	(Cr 72)
Cunningham and Jeffree (1975)	(Cu & J 75)
Cunningham and Sloper (1977)	(Cu & Sl 77)
Dodd (1975)	(D 75)
Edlund (1971)	(Ed 71)
Evans (1977)	(E 77)
Ferber, Keeley and Shemberg (1974)	(F, K & Sh 74)
Filler (1976)	(F 76)
Fink and Bice-Gray (1979)	(F & B.G 79)
Frisch and Schumaker (1974)	(Fr & Sch 74)
Fritsch, Fritsch and Pechstein (1976)	(F, F, & P 76)

TABLE 2.1 (continued)

CODE FOR INTERVENTION AND SURVEY STUDIES REVIEWED

Author/Authors, Date	Code
Galloway and Galloway (1971)	(G & G 71)
Gath (1977)	(Ga 77)
Gayton and Walker (1974)	(G & W 74)
Golden, Hermine and Pashayan (1976)	(Go, H & P 76)
Hall, Axelrod, Tyler et al (1972)	(H, Ax, & T 72)
Heifetz (1977)	(H 77)
Hemsley, Howlin, Berger et al (1978)	(H, H, B 78)
Herbert and Baer (1972)	(H & Ba 72)
Herbert, Pinkston, Hayden et al (1973)	(H, P, H 73)
Hewson (1977)	(Hew 77)
Jacobson, Bernal and Lopes (1973)	(Ja, B & L 73)
Jeffree and McConkey (1974)	(J & Mc 74)
Jeffree, McConkey et al (1976)	(J, & Mc 76)
Latham and Hofmeister (1973)	(L & H 73)
Lovaas, Koegel, Simmons and Long (1973)	(L, K, S & L 73)
MacDonald, Blott, Gordon et al (1974)	(Mac, B, G 74)
Mash, Lazere, Terdal, and Garner (1973)	(M, L, T & G 73)
Mash and Terdal (1973)	(M & T 73)
Miller and Sloane (1976)	(M & Sl 76)
Myers and Warkany (1977)	(M & W 77)
O'Kelly-Collard (1978)	(O'K-C 78)
Peine and Munro (1973)	(P & M 73)
Prior (1977)	(Pr 77)

TABLE 2.1 (continued)

CODE FOR INTERVENTION AND SURVEY STUDIES REVIEWED

Author/Authors, Date	Code
Revill and Blunden (1979)	(R & Bl 79)
Ribes-Inesta, Duran, Evans et al (1973)	(RI, D, E 73)
Rose (1974b)	(R 74b)
Ross and Ross (1979)	(R & R 79)
Sailor (1971)	(S 71)
Sajwaj (1973)	(Saj 73)
Salzinger, Feldman and Portnoy (1970)	Sa, F & P 70)
Sandow and Clarke (1978)	(S & Cl 78)
Seitz and Riedell (1974)	(S & R 74)
Skelton (1972)	(Sk 72)
Snyder and McLean (1976)	(Sn & Mc 76)
Sommers and Starkey (1977)	(S & St 77)
Sosne, Handleman and Harris (1979)	(S, H & H 79)
Sparrow and Zigler (1978)	(Sp & Z 78)
Stone (1973)	(St 73)
Stone and Chesney (1978)	(St & Ch 78)
Strain (1975)	(Str 75)
Striefel and Wetherby (1973)	(Str & W 73)
Tavormina, Hampson and Luscomb (1976)	(T, H & L 76)
Tein (1977)	(T 77)
Urban (1978)	(U 78)
Wehman and Marchant (1978)	(We & M 78)
Wheeler and Sulzer (1970)	(W & S 70)
Whitman, Zakaras and Chardos (1971)	(W, Z & Ch 71)

TABLE 2.2

DESCRIPTION OF STUDIES REVIEWED: TIME PERIOD

OF SURVEY OR INTERVENTION: DETAILS OF SUBJECTS

Code	Description of Studies
(A, G, A & S. 77)	Survey of effects of parent attitudes to diagnosis and service provision for the intellectually handicapped: 215 families, children under 6 years of age.
(B & B. 73)	Contingency contracting for parents to enable them to modify their pre-school children's speech: 6 families, 7 weeks interaction.
(Ben. 73)	Examination of alternative forms of teaching and therapy on the motor, perceptual, verbal and social skills development of the mildly retarded.
(B. 76)	Testing speech imitation skills of 108 subjects over 2½ months. Mean C.A. 11 yrs 4 mths.
(B. M & M. 77)	Observation and analysis of a mother's communication with her Down's syndrom child aged 2 years. 4 months.
(Be. 74)	Counselling of parents and behaviour in modification training for one child for 4 months with follow up. C.A. 7 yrs.
(B. S. & M. 78)	Examination of verbally initiated social interactions using a scan sampling technique: 200 children, Age range 2 yrs. 3 mths to 17 yrs. 5 mths.
(Bi, Br & G. 75)	Teaching behaviour modification techniques to mothers of 16 D.S. children for 6 months. Mean C.A. 2 yrs.
(Bu & P. 73)	Parents teaching their retarded child to chew solid food: 28 day programme. C.A. 8 yrs.
(Cl-R. 76)	Operant language training programme for 28

TABLE 2.2. (continued)

DESCRIPTION OF STUDIES REVIEWED: TIME PERIOD

OF SURVEY OR INTERVENTION: DETAILS OF SUBJECTS

Code	Description of Studies
	children for 10 weeks but continuing. Age range 3 mths. to 3 yrs. 7 mths.
(C.M. & R. 74)	Facilitating the cognitive and speech development of up to 50 pre-school children - early comparative results 1 year's intervention.
(C.M. & R. 79)	Language and cognitive developments of pre-school children after 5 years of intervention in clinic or classroom. 60 subjects.
(Cr 72)	Assessing language structure, knowledge and learning ability of 31 retarded subjects. Age range 7 yrs. 1 mth. to 16 yrs. 6 mths.
(Cu & J. 75)	Tutor workshops for parents to develop their children's self help and speech skills. 36 families for 10 weeks - 5 meetings. Age range 6 months to 6 years.
(Cu. & Sl 77)	Process of professional and parent contact for 47 families with D.S. children.
(D. 75)	Ability of D.S. and non D.S. retarded children to recognise, remember and reproduce words. 20 children. Mean C.A. 9 years.
(Ed. 71)	Training parents and teachers to reinforce children's school assignments at school and at home in order to improve the children's participation in classroom activities. Intervention from 18 days to almost one school year - 6 subjects aged 16 yrs (N=1) 6 yrs (N=2) & 11 yrs (N=3)
(E. 77)	Defining the distinct language abilities of D.S. children by factors analysis of the "general language factor". 101 D.S. children. Age range 8 yrs. to 21 yrs.

TABLE 2.2 (continued)

DESCRIPTION OF STUDIES REVIEWED: TIME PERIOD

OF SURVEY OR INTERVENTION: DETAILS OF SUBJECTS

Code	Description of Studies
(F, K, & Sh. 74)	Behaviour modification training for parents to help them improve their children's social behaviour. 7 families for 3 mths. Age range 5 yrs. to 10 yrs.
(F. 76)	Teaching mothers to organise/modify their teaching. 21 subjects over 3 weeks. Mean C.A. 3 yrs. 6 mths.
(F. & B. G. 79)	A comparison of two different teaching strategies on the ability to acquire and recall five two syllable functional sight words by 10 subjects for 1 mth. Mean C.A. 4 yrs. 6 mths.
(Fr. & Sch. 74)	Use of reinforcement procedures to train correct use of receptive preposition for 3 children for 2 months. Ages 3 yrs. 5 mths, 4 yrs. and 11 yrs.
(F, F, & P. 76)	Mothers' ability to cope with home based teaching: Evaluation of the influence of measures of self image, social situation, attitudes to children for 69 families with pre-schoolers.
(G, & G. 71)	Reducing the rocking and improving the attending behaviour of a 7 year old with P.K.U. over 4 months.
(Ga. 77)	Comparison of parents coping skills: Parents, Down's syndrome children and normal children. New born babies. 6 interviews for 30 families over 2 years.

37

TABLE 2.2 (continued)

DESCRIPTION OF STUDIES REVIEWED: TIME PERIOD

OF SURVEY OR INTERVENTION: DETAILS OF SUBJECTS

Code	Description of Studies
(G. & W. 74)	Survey of when parents were told about Down's Syndrome. 85 familes. Mean C.A. 10 years.
(G., H & P. 76)	Survey of parents' level of education and their children's mental development for 109 families. Age range 3 yrs. 10 mths to 16 years.
(H, Ax, & T. 72)	Social reinforcement to shape self help behaviour for 4 children for 2 months. Ages from 4 yrs. to 10 years.
(H. 77)	Use of behaviour modification manuals and professional assistance in facilitating self help & language skills. 160 families for 20 weeks. 2-14 yrs.
(H, H, B. 78)	Family treatment by home visits for 16 autistic children for 6 months. Mean C.A. 6 yrs. 2 mths.
(H. & Ba. 72)	Parents recording their attention for appropriate child behaviour to improve their children's attention span, social interaction and speech. 2 children for 6 months, both S.s aged 5 years.
(H, P, H. 73)	Teaching a mother to modify her son's aggressive behaviour. 45 hours intervention. Age 4 yrs.
(Hew. 77)	Weekly parent meetings to train parents to develop children's self help and speech skills. 12 weekly meetings, 31 families. Mean C.A. of children, 8 yrs. 7 mths.
(Ja, B & L. 73)	Improving child language by using reinforcement procedures to teach non-verbal concepts. 1 subject for 5 weeks, aged 17 years.
(J. & Mc. 74)	Extending language through structured play for 1 child for 4 weeks (20 sessions). Age 3 yrs.

TABLE 2.2 (continued)

DESCRIPTION OF STUDIES REVIEWED: TIME PERIOD

OF SURVEY OR INTERVENTION: DETAILS OF SUBJECTS

Code   Description of Studies

(J. & Mc. 76)   Training developmental skills to children and
                       childrens gemes to their parents. 2 yr project.
                       Average time of parent involvement 6 mths. C.A. 2-5yrs

(L. & H. 73)   Training parents to develop self help and
                       pre-speech skills by means of a multi-media
                       training package for 40 families for 2 weeks.
                       Age range from 2 years to 6 years.

(L, K, S & L. 73)   Long term study and follow up of the appropriate
                       and inappropriate behaviours of 20 autistic
                       children after treatment for 12 to 14 months.
                       Age from 4 years to 6½ years.

(Mac, B, G. 74)   Behaviour modification training for parents to
                       develop two word utterances for 3 Down's syndrome
                       children over 5 months. Age range 3 yrs. to
                       5 yrs.

(M, L, T & G. 73)   Training four parents to achieve compliance to
                       commands by their children by means of approp-
                       riate social reinforcement. 10 weeks. Ages
                       from 4 years to 9 years.

(M. & T. 73)   Group training for ten mothers to develop their
                       children's play. 10 one hour sessions. Age
                       range from 4 years to 10 years.

(M. & Sl. 76)   Parent training effects on children's speech.
                       5 children for 4 months. Age range 6 to 12 yrs.

(M. & W. 77)   Social work counselling, physiotherapy and
                       occupational therapy to develop self help and
                       play skills for 6 children for 8 weeks. Ages
                       2½ to 3 years.

TABLE 2.2 (continued)

DESCRIPTION OF STUDIES REVIEWED: TIME PERIOD

OF SURVEY OR INTERVENTION: DETAILS OF SUBJECTS

Code	Description of Studies
(O'K-C. 78)	Examination of maternal linguistic environments for 6 Down's syndrome and 6 normal children. Mean C.A. for Down's syndrome = 3 yrs. 2 mths., Normal = 1 yrs. 6 mths.
(P. & M. 73)	Behaviour management training by means of classes reading and home assignments. 47 familes for 5 weeks. Pre-school age and lower grade primary children.
(Pr. 77)	Comparisons of the language abilities of 20 autistic and 20 retarded children. Mean C.A. Autistic = 11 yrs. 5 mths. Other Retarded = 11 yrs. 8 mths.
(R. & Bl 79)	Home training procedures by clinical psychologists to develop mother and language skills for 19 subjects over 8 months. C.A. age range from 8 months to 4 years.
(Rl, D, E. 73)	Dispersing tokens in a social setting in order to teach four brain damaged children to make controlled physical contact with adults. 50 half hour sessions over 5 weeks. C.A. range from 5 to 14 years.
(R. 74b)	Behaviour modification for parents to facilitate their children's language and social behaviour. 33 families for 10 weeks. Age range from 3 yrs. to 8 years.
(R. & R. 79)	Training the selective attention skills of E.M.R. children for six weeks. 40 subjects Mean C.A. 8 yrs. 4 mths.
(S. 71)	Training parents to reduce/eliminate undesirable child behaviour. 4 families over 4 months.

TABLE 2.2 (continued)

DESCRIPTION OF STUDIES REVIEWED: TIME PERIOD

OF SURVEY OR INTERVENTION: DETAILS OF SUBJECTS

Code	Description of Studies
(Saj. 73)	Training parents to reduce undesirable child behaviour. 4 families over 4 months.
(Sa, F & P. 70)	Behaviour modification of self help behaviour for 8 families over 2 years. Ages 3 to 12 years.
(S & Cl. 78)	Home based intervention to develop self help and pre-speech skills for 32 families for 3 years. Age range 18 mths. to 3 yrs. 4 mths.
(S. & R. 74)	Modifying a mother's utterances to facilitate her child's verbalisations. 1 child for 8 weeks. Age 4 years.
(Sk. 72)	Identifying parents' difficulties in coping with their retarded children. 90 children in institutions, 38 at home. Mean C.A. 5 years.
(Sn & Mc. 76)	Use of selective listening, the establishment of joint reference and feed back mechanisms in children's language acquisition strategies.
(S. & St. 77)	Factors relating to differences in verbal communication skills of 29 Down's syndrome children. Age range 7 to 19 years, and 20 non-retarded children, age range 3 to 5 yrs.
(S, H & H. 79)	A six stage behaviour modification programme for teaching functional self initiated speech to autistic type children.
(Sp. & Z. 78)	Comparison of interventions to evaluate effects of patterning on motor and pre-speech skills. One year for 15 subjects.

TABLE 2.2 (continued)

DESCRIPTION OF STUDIES REVIEWED: TIME PERIOD

OF SURVEY OR INTERVENTION: DETAILS OF SUBJECTS

Code	Description of Studies
(St. 73)	Survey of medical/social/emotional needs of 31 families with Down's syndrome children. Age range 5 months to 11 years.
(St. & Ch 78)	Survey of attachment behaviours' of retarded infants'. 15 mothers and their children for one year.
(Str. 75)	Presentation of social dramatic activities to increase the social play exhibited by eight retarded pre-schoolers for 1 month. Age range 4 years to 4 years 4 months.
(Str. & W. 73)	Teaching motor responses to verbal instructions for 1 subject for 3 months. Age 11 years.
(T, H, & L. 76)	Parents evaluating the effects of behaviour and reflective counselling on children's social development. 45 mothers for 8 weeks.
(T. 77)	General description of intervention services that could be provided for handicapped or disadvantaged pre-schoolers.
(U. 78)	Description of ongoing provision of early intervention services for at risk pre-schoolers.
(We. & M. 78)	Behaviour management programmes to reduce inappropriate object contact. Time sampling procedure for 5 days. C.A. 7 years.
(W. & S. 70)	Training a subject to use sentence forms that include articles and verbs for 7 weeks - 38 half hour sessions. C.A. 8 years.
(W, Z & Ch. 71)	Teaching motor responses to verbal instructions for 2 children for 2 months. Age 4½ yrs. and 7 years.

(1979) for their lack of base-line data, for their lack of regular weekly or fortnightly contact with their subjects or for their general descriptions of language attainment. Yet the study did last for 5 years. It does record that some groups of intellectually handicapped children made only small progress, and it does make comparisons of the receptive and expressive language skills of different groups of children which parents can comprehend.

CHARACTERISTICS OF INTERVENTION PROGRAMMES

Table 2.3 identifies characteristics of some intervention programmes that have taken place in the 1970's. Forty-six per cent report standardised data in the form of either language ages, measured IQ scores or formal descriptions related to standardised data of the degree and nature of subjects' intellectual handicap. Eighty-four per cent make use of criterion referenced data thus confirming the importance attached to behaviour modification programmes. However, only thirty per cent of studies make use of both standardised and criterion reference data. Twenty-four per cent report the statistical adjustment of data in order to evaluate treatment or other effects. Yet, this should not be regarded as too great a criticism for so many of the interventions reported are single case studies which have few needs for statistical adjustments. Seventy per cent make use of controls in the form of comparison with no treatment groups, or of staggered entry into a treatment programme or via the use of carefully gathered baseline data. Fifty per cent assess the reliability of parent or teacher observations or make specific reference to this reliability factor. This is important in parent based programmes because of the need for parents and the therapists to be as realistic as possible about a child's achievements. Seventy-four per cent make comparisons with other studies in their evaluation of the effectiveness of their programmes. However, only twenty-six per cent report or make reference to the generalisation of skills in different environments and only twenty-five per cent of the studies report follow-up data or report that a follow-up is planned. Generalisation of skills and follow-up after the termination of the initial intervention are factors that concern parents. "Will the skill my child has acquired generalise to other situations?" and . . . "Will you be organising another teaching programme after this one has finished?" or indeed, "When can I see you again?" are recurrent questions for parents. However, in the history of intervention programmes, the factors of generalisation and follow-up do represent secondary goals. The initial goal for so many families must be to get some intervention established, and concentrating on factors such as generalisation and follow-up may hinder, or be seen to hinder the establishment of intervention in the first place.

PARENT VARIABLES WHICH MIGHT DETERMINE THE SUCCESS OF AN INTERVENTION PROGRAMME

There is clearly no guarantee, that merely training parents in the use of play, in developmental speech therapy techniques, or in the principles of structured teaching and behaviour modification, that there can be an effective application of these principles. Certainly, parent involvement would appear to be so much more effective than the therapist operating in an isolated clinic or school and therefore never being able to directly observe that vital parent-child interaction in its natural environment (Hawkins et al., 1966). However, there are many other parent variables that need to be taken account of in any evaluation of a parent oriented intervention programme. For example, Golden, Hermine and Pashayan (1976) demonstrate that longer formal post-secondary education by parents resulted in the measured IQ scores of their children being higher than for those children whose parents had no post-secondary education. They recommend that the level of education of parents with intellectually handicapped children be part of intake information. If necessary, in cases where the parents' formal education is limited, a more vigorous programme could be considered and, if possible, implemented for their children at an early age. However, according to Cunningham and Jeffree (1975) and Salzinger,

TABLE 2.3

CHARACTERISTICS OF INTERVENTION PROGRAMMES

CODE	1	2	3	4	5	6	7	8
(B. & B. 73)		√				√	√	
(Ben. 73)		√		√		√	√	
(B, M & M. 77)	√	√			√	√		
(Be,74)		√		√				√
(Bi, Br & G. 75)	√		√			√		
(Bu. & P. 73)		√		√			√	
(Cl-R. 76)	√	√				√		
(C, M & R. 74)	√			√				√
(C, M & R. 79)	√			√				√
(Cr. 72)	√	√				√		
(Cu. & J. 75)	√			√		√		√
(Ed. 71)		√		√		√		
(F, K, & Sh. 74)		√			√	√		
(Fi. 76)	√	√	√	√	√	√		
(F, & B-G. 79)	√	√	√		√			
(Fr. & Sch. 74)		√		√	√	√		
(G. & G. 71)		√		√				
(G. 77)		√		√		√	√	
(H, Ax & T. 72)		√	√	√	√	√		
(H. & Ba. 72)		√		√	√	√		√

KEY
1. Reporting of Formal Standardised Data.
2. Reporting of Criterion Reference Data.
3. Statistical adjusting of data for evaluating the effects of treatment.
4. Use of Controls: no treatment or staggered entry into programme or baseline data.
5. Assessing the reliability of parents'/teachers'/observations.
6. Comparison with other studies.
7. Examination and Reporting of generalisation across stimulus settings.
8. Report of follow-up to examine long term effects of treatment.

TABLE 2.3 (continued)

CHARACTERISTICS OF INTERVENTION PROGRAMMES

CODE	1	2	3	4	5	6	7	8
(H, P & H. 73)		√	√	√	√	√		
(Ja, B & L. 73)	√	√		√			√	
(J & Mc. 74)		√		√	√	√		
(J. & Mc. 76)	√	√			√			
(L. & H. 73)		√	√	√				√
(L, K, S & L. 73)	√	√	√	√	√	√	√	√
(Mac, B & G. 74)		√			√	√	√	
(M, L, T & G. 73)		√			√	√		
(M. & T. 73)	√	√		√	√			
(M. & Sl. 76)		√		√	√	√	√	
(M. & W. 77)		√				√		
(O'K-C. 78)	√	√	√			√		
(P. & M. 73)		√		√		√		
(R. & Bl. 79)	√	√		√		√		
(R-I, D, E. 73)		√		√	√	√		
(R. 74b)	√	√				√		
(R. & R. 79)	√		√	√	√	√		
(S. 71)		√		√	√	√	√	
(Saj. 73)		√		√		√	√	
(Sa, F & P. 70)		√	√	√	√			
(S. & Cl. 78)	√		√	√	√	√		√

KEY

1. Reporting of Formal Standardised Data.
2. Reporting of Criterion Reference Data.
3. Statistical adjusting of data for evaluating the effects of treatment.
4. Use of Controls: no treatment or staggered entry into programme or baseline data.
5. Assessing the reliability of parents'/teachers'/observations.
6. Comparison with other studies.
7. Examination and Reporting of generalisation across stimulus settings.
8. Report of follow-up to examine long term effects of treatment.

TABLE 2.3 (continued)

CHARACTERISTICS OF INTERVENTION PROGRAMMES

CODE	1	2	3	4	5	6	7	8
(S. & R. 74)		√			√	√		√
(S, H & H. 79)	√	√		√	√		√	
(S. & Z. 78)	√		√	√		√		
(Str. 75)	√	√		√	√	√	√	
(T, H & L. 76)		√		√		√		
(U. 78)	√	√				√		
(W. & M. 78)		√		√				
(W. & S. 70)		√		√	√	√	√	√
(W, Z & Ch. 71)	√			√	√	√		
TOTAL	23	42	12	35	25	37	12	10
% of Studies	46	84	24	70	50	74	26	25

KEY

1. Reporting of Formal Standardised Data.
2. Reporting of Criterion Reference Data.
3. Statistical adjusting of data for evaluating the effects of treatment.
4. Use of Controls: no treatment or staggered entry into programme or baseline data.
5. Assessing the reliability of parents'/teachers'/observations.
6. Comparison with other studies.
7. Examination and Reporting of generalisation across stimulus settings.
8. Report of follow-up to examine long term effects of treatment.

Feldman and Portnoy (1970), educational levels did not appear to affect the parents' performances in training their children.

Reference has already been made to the parental acceptance or adjustment to having an intellectually handicapped child. However, few differences in attitude appear between parents of children with different forms of intellectual handicap. Johnson and Olley (1971) review the literature comparing the achievements of Down's syndrome and non-Down's syndrome children on a variety of behavioural tasks, but again no attempt is made here to include the vital variable of parents' attitude. Hood, Shank and Williamson (1948) tried to correlate attitudes and personal traits of mothers with a general index of speech proficiency in cerebral palsied children living in their home environment. The results are statistically not conclusive but are similar to the findings of Lawrence (1972) where there were indications that ability by parents to accept slow progress, self-sufficiency and emotional stability tended to favour better language development in their children. Peeters (1978), in a cross cultural study, demonstrates the relationship between maternal attitudes and the obtaining of services for autistic children. The more open and innovative mother is observed to gain considerably more comprehensive services than the more defensive and less innovative mother. However, few have systematically gathered information about parental attitude to teaching their children, largely, it would appear, through lack of sensitive instrumentation. Hill (1976) and Johnson (1975) made comprehensive use of Strom's Parent Attitude Inventory (Strom and Slaughter, 1976), in evaluating the relationship between parents' expressed attitudes and parents' observed behaviour, in their interaction with their children. Burden (1977) stresses the need to take account of maternal attitudes in evaluating intervention projects with severely handicapped children, but once again this appears as a recommendation rather than an example of the effects of parent attitudes on teaching.

Other parent variables which may determine parents' success in teaching are the length and intensity of parental involvement. Yet there are very few long term studies which evaluate the effectiveness of programmes from the point of view of length of parental involvement (see Table 2.2.). The nature of parental involvement may likewise determine a programme's success. Eyeberg and Johnson's (1974) paper found that contingency contracting was superior to all other measures of commencing and maintaining parental involvement. Similarly, Hirsch and Walder (1969) found that they could use a refundable deposit system to increase parent motivation and maintain a one hundred per cent attendance at all group meetings. Yet both papers say little about parental success in teaching their children, or comment on the importance of group cohesion as effective means of maintaining parental involvement. It would appear that contracts similar to those of Hirsch and Walder are only effective in the short term when parents are able quickly to recognise improvement in their children's skills as a result of intervention.

CONCLUSION

A lifetime's work and definite alterations to a family's domestic life confront parents of the intellectually handicapped. This is even more so when they become involved in intervention programmes. Language intervention programmes are particularly sought by parents because they are considered to help maximise social interaction. Yet we need to know which professionals should be involved and what should be the function, content and goals of such programmes. When should an intervention programme begin and how long should it last? What factors are most likely to determine its success or failure? The literature answers some questions while other questions require further examination and research. Clearly, intervention of some form should begin, if possible as soon as the child is born. However, the evidence is quite inconclusive that effective interventions are age specific, though the tendency is to emphasise that maximum benefits accrue in interventions with infants and young children.

Evidence exists that optimum teaching occurs when close attention is given to relating a highly structured programme to the needs of the developing child, and in particular, to relating the child's growing physical skills to both his receptive and expressive language. Parents of the intellectually handicapped recognise that teaching procedures for their children are similar to those used for normal children. Yet for parents to develop their children's skills, their teaching needs to be applied with a precision and regularity which often disrupts household routines and which, unless the child is clearly observed to be improving, cannot be (or are not) maintained over months and years. This time period is so necessary for skills taught to generalise to other settings. Parent attitude to the intellectually handicapped child is a key variable in effective intervention in the short and long term. Attitudes can be guided and shaped, provided an unobtrusive and non-threatening means can be devised of monitoring these parent attitudes.

Contracts between parent and professional may appear to work well in the short term. Yet sustaining home based teaching over many years, if not a child's lifetime, requires a cohesive face-to-face support service which itself not only provides effective teaching methods but recognises and uses parent hopes, ingenuity, imagination and stamina, and allays frustrations. At the heart of this is a trust and confidence between parent and therapist. The support service is based on the recognition that parents wish to do something themselves for their children, but that equally, if they are left alone, they can become discouraged, frustrated, defensive and less open to suggestions about teaching skills that parent and teacher, and parent and therapist *together* can create and sustain.

Parents of the severely handicapped are often afraid for their child's future. That is the nature of their imagination given their circumstances. Yet parents advance their own and their children's skills because of their engagement in intervention programmes. The personal commitment of parents to develop their skills, to harness their intellectual and emotional commitment, can only result in enhancing their child's future. Services from Education, Health and Welfare, and dissemination of continuing research at the face-to-face level of parents and therapists, can support, sustain and develop parents' commitment.

Chapter Three

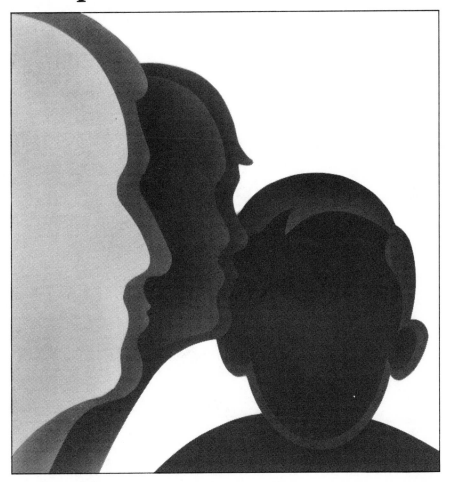

Parent Involvement —
The Language Teaching Programme

INTRODUCTION

It is clear that the content of so-called "expert" advice on child rearing changes with fashion. Stendler (1950), in her historical survey, demonstrated that much of the factual basis for this "expert" advice is obscure, and that much of the rest is theory. Sometimes this theory is a product of keen observation and closely reasoned thought. Yet it is seldom buttressed by carefully gathered, rigorously evaluated, empirical data. A long-term parent training programme requires empirical evidence for its inception and continuation. The literature indicates the focus on behaviour modification and single case studies. These studies stress the importance of criterion referenced data as a basis for reliable and realistic teaching. In this programme the ideal teaching situation, as indicated by the literature, had to be blended with what was possible and realistic for parents and therapists.

During the initial interviews with parents, information was obtained about the nature of the language problem which each intellectually handicapped child displayed. This information was supported by the evidence obtained during the initial diagnosis in Stage I (Rees 1978), (see also Figure 3.1 p. 54). As such, the rationale for developing such a parent-oriented language teaching programme reflects both parents' wishes and an evaluation of current research. The rationale takes account of:

(i) *Optimising parent-child interaction*

Parent interactions with their children are the *source* of their attitudes and values. It is these attitudes and values which will help them to cope or not cope with the stress of having an intellectually handicapped child. However, these attitudes and values change over the developmental period and are as likely to result from *interaction* with the child rather than to be based on responses to intellectual handicap *per se*. Therefore, a parent training programme provides an opportunity to facilitate optimal parent-child interaction.

(ii) *Parents as models for their children*

Parents' behaviour is so often imitated by children. For example, there is recent verification that very young infants may imitate specific acts of adults (Maratos 1973; Uzgiris 1974). Furthermore, this imitation could also be expected by intellectually handicapped children. As such, parents need to be made as aware as possible of their modelling role and of the importance of optimum models for imitation with even the most severely handicapped child. Of particular relevance here is Trevarthen's (1977) evidence of clear cases of specific imitation by neonates of such behaviours as tongue protrusion, mouth opening, head movement and smiling. There is a need, therefore, for parents to *be aware of* what behaviours are imitated and which of these are most relevant in the development of an ongoing *communication system* between them and their intellectually handicapped children.

(iii) *Critical periods of development and shared understandings*

For various language skills there are "critical periods" when the mother can best facilitate their onset. Therefore, by utilizing the concept of the "critical period" of mother-child interaction, it may be possible to shape the child's reactions. For example, Prechtl (1958) suggests that certain behavioural patterns in the infant are prerequisites for a mothering response in human mothers. Hofsten and Lindhagen (1979) demonstrate how and when infants come to master visually directed reaching. This information is, of course, most relevant in the effective teaching by parents of certain receptive language skills to the intellectually handicapped. Ackerman (1979) demonstrates that at certain ages children can begin to interpret definite descriptions or have the ability to infer a speaker's intent in making a referential statement.

These studies demonstrate that such relevant language behaviours as the directed head turning response, the instinctive responses on the part of the baby of crying, smiling, following and clinging (Bowlby 1958), the skill in reaching for objects, and children's understanding of definite descriptions, do tend to occur at certain "critical periods" in their lives. However, if these and allied behaviours by the child fail to occur, or occur developmentally much later, then mothers may fail to develop the relevant reaction. It may be necessary therefore for these relevant maternal reactions to be programmed and planned for, rather than their absence lamented.

It is helpful to parents to understand the quite sophisticated nature of the communication between them and their intellectually handicapped children. For example, once a communication dialogue has been established between an intellectually handicapped child and his parents (even a dialogue of gesture), then it is highly likely that it *could* evolve further towards elaboration of more and more sophisticated *shared* understandings. Evidence exists that the success of the communication system is dependent on the behaviour of *both* parent and child.

This evidence suggests that it requires only one of the partners to be insensitive to signals for the communication sequence to break down. Therefore, any lack of responsiveness by intellectually handicapped children would make it more difficult for their mothers to keep up the kind of active information dialogue in which most mothers engage their children. In this way, the intellectually handicapped child cannot initiate parents' responses that enrich the environment for himself or herself. Hence there is an apparent need to support parents and to produce a training programme which is sensitive to particular children's needs, and which takes into account the complex forms of communication and understanding that could evolve.

Bateson (1971) has written about the succession of addresses and replies between parent and child. These succeed one another in a temporal configuration of behaviour remarkably like that of a conversation between adults. Bateson has described such behaviour as "proto-conversational". Accordingly, an aim of the present parent training programme was to construct teaching situations that were, or could become, proto-conversational in the sense that they constituted a succession of requests and replies between parent and child. Parents felt that these language behaviours could be developed and utilized in the home setting.

(iv) *The linguist's contribution*

From a linguistic point of view, the development of an intellectually handicapped child's language also involves joint action. From the start, the intellectually handicapped child is equipped with some communication procedures for eliciting help from others. Bruner (1975) often calls this the *demand mode.* Many of these procedures for eliciting help are derived from innate patterns of expressing discomfort that activate adults. By the third or fourth month of the normal baby's life, most mothers claim to be able to distinguish several forms of demand calling, and though these can be distinguished phonologically, they are heavily dependent on context for interpretation. Even for the intellectually handicapped, it appears that demand cries of this kind are insistent, have a wide spectrum acoustically, and show no pauses in anticipation of response. Bruner (1975) describes the development of joint parent-child action patterns: the *demand mode*, then the *request mode,* then the *exchange mode*, and lastly the *reciprocal mode.* It is at the stage of the reciprocal mode (from ten months onwards in the normal child) that interactions between parent and child can be organised around a task that possesses "exteriority, constraint and division of labour".

At the reciprocal stage, structured receptive language tasks become most relevant. In these tasks, the parent and child enter upon a task with reciprocal, though non-identical, roles. The receptive language task and its constituent acts and objects (see Appendix II) become the focus of joint attention and anticipation. Increasingly, even with the most handicapped, gestures and most vocalization become associated with specific tasks or predictable actions. However, this joint action in the learning of communication skills can only be acquired if there is a consistent caretaker who is preferably a caring parent. A variety of studies point to the importance of this consistent caretaker role in order that linguistic competence may be developed (Sander *et al.*, 1970; Ainsworth 1975).

(v) *The child's future status*

There is evidence (Myers 1978) that improved communication skills, both inside and outside the home, improve the status of the intellectually handicapped. If communication skills could be improved, then parents feel that their children could become more involved in social life. As such, this contribution would lead to improvement in status. Indeed, when the social status of these children is at its lowest — the *pariah* status, according to Hanks and Hanks (1948) — then they have fewer rights and are so often seen by the majority of the population as a threat. This can cause unnecessary stress for parents. A parent training programme, especially one initiated by parents, may reduce parent stress. For many parents there is an ever-present attitude that the problem of their child's intellectual handicap is likely to, or indeed does, dominate their emotional lives. This is so unless they have been given quite specific help from professionals and others.

For example, over fifty per cent of parents in the present study indicated that in order to protect themselves they frequently withdrew from social life, so that they would be protected, as one parent expressed it, "from the comments, the gratuitous advice, the criticisms and reactions of others". This withdrawal can be seen to intensify feelings of isolation, shock and disappointment. They may withdraw from physiotherapy and speech therapy services, and social work visits. Where these are available and participated in regularly they could prevent the entrenching of attitudes and defensiveness which is an obstacle to parent innovation. It is of course these services that for some parents may be a constant reminder of their child's difference from others. Yet there is also evidence (Kimber and Porritt 1976) that parents' use of these services is likely to make them more innovative and persistent in teaching their children.

(vi) *Co-ordination of services*

If parents are to provide consistent care and teaching then they need support from professionals in the field (*Special Educational Needs* 1978, Ch. 9). Professionals, such as speech therapists, occupational therapists, physiotherapists, counsellors and teachers, were already working with the families in this sample (see below p. 58). A parent-oriented training programme provided the opportunity for co-ordination of these services.

THE LANGUAGE TEACHING PROGRAMME

The *Parents as Language Therapists for Intellectually Handicapped Children* programme covers a period of almost three years. It was organised in three stages:

STAGE I   Preparation and production of language programme.

STAGE II   Training and teaching.

STAGE III Support services and termination.

Evaluation of these services took place throughout each of these stages. The diagram below, Figure 3.1, illustrates the stages, content and form of the *Parents as Language Therapists* programme. Each stage is described in turn.

STAGE I — Preparation of Parents and Production of the Language Programme

These activities follow in sequence.

(a) *Standardised Language and Intelligence Quotient Assessment*

In order to write and produce the language programme at the conclusion of Stage I, it was necessary to assess the levels of verbal functioning and, where possible, the levels of measured intelligence, of this heterogeneous sample (see Tables 1.1, 1.2, 1.3 and Fig. 1.1). The language scales chosen for this purpose were the Reynell Developmental Language Scales (Reynell, 1969b), and for the assessment of IQ, the revised Stanford Binet (Form LM).

The Reynell Language Scales have a developmental orientation. According to Reynell, they cover the important developmental stages from the very beginning of language until school age. In particular, they enable the receptive and expressive aspects of language to be

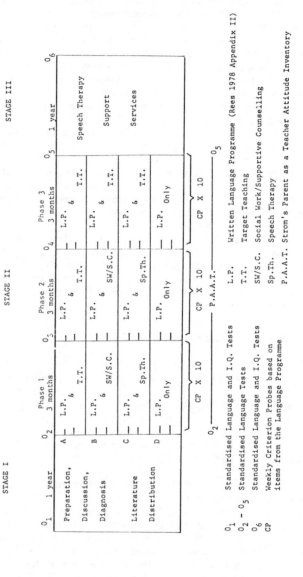

Figure 3.1

RESEARCH DESIGN

DIAGRAM TO ILLUSTRATE STAGES AND CONTENT
OF THE LANGUAGE TEACHING PROGRAMME

54

assessed separately. The Reynell Language Scales also served the need of this research because the tests were developed in a clinical setting and used as a clinical tool throughout their development (Reynell, 1969b). Accordingly, each child was tested, and receptive and expressive language ages in months were computed, and, where at all possible, each child was assessed on the revised Stanford Binet (Form LM) (Terman and Merrill 1961).

(b) *Descriptive information from Parents*

Once standardised language testing had been completed, this was followed by the collection of descriptive information from parents about their family situation. Answers related to the following were collected in individual open-ended interviews:

(i) Family size and position of the handicapped child in the family;
(ii) Parental and sibling reaction to the handicapped child;
(iii) Parents' views about the language levels of their handicapped child and parents' knowledge of factors which help determine language acquisition;
(iv) Parents' expectations for their children;
(v) Chances of parents carrying out regular language teaching on a daily basis and parents' attitude towards such teaching.

(c) *Diagnosis*

This diagnosis took the form of:

(i) Parents responding to specific statements relating to their child's language ability (see Appendix IV). The specific language statements were derived from a search of the literature (Bayley, 1970; Crabtree, 1969; Frankenburg and Dodds, 1970; Lerea, 1958; Sheridan, 1964; Templin, 1967; Uzgiris and Hunt, 1975). They are divided into seven levels with approximately twenty statements for each level. Parents were presented with only those levels which were considered relevant for their child. Parents' responses to these statements were examined for later inclusion in the development of the language manual *Parents as Language Therapists for Intellectually Handicapped children* (Rees 1978, Appendix II). The principal aim of these "language statements" was to *begin* to involve parents in assessing their child's language development.

(ii) Parents observed their child receiving language teaching at a level relevant to his ability. This was done to give an initial demonstration to the parent of the nature of language teaching on an individual basis. Parents either observed the child through a one-way screen or sat in the same room alongside the teacher/therapist.

(iii) Parents were videotaped interacting with their child in either a children's nursery playroom equipped with large and small toys and reading material, or in a 2m by 2m clinic teaching room generally devoid of equipment except for the stimulus toys/pictures being used. The videotapes were then played back and discussed with the parents to try to establish:

(a) the most suitable conditions in which to work;
(b) whether these conditions were available in the home;
(c) the optimum length of a language therapy session;
(d) factors which might determine the optimum length of a language therapy session;
(e) the most suitable teaching materials to be used;
(f) the particular techniques related to gaining and sustaining attention that could be used.

(d) *Literature Distribution and Home Visits*

Group meetings, individual family interviews and diagnosis established that parents needed to be given much more information about all aspects of language development and teaching. Accordingly, during the middle of Stage I, (Fig. 3.1 p. 54), literature was distributed to parents by either health visitors from the Capital Territory Health Commission or by qualified teachers undertaking postgraduate studies in Special Education. The literature distribution took the form of printed handouts presented under the following headings:

(i) Positions for Feeding to Encourage Normal Swallowing.
(ii) Exercises for Chewing and Swallowing.
(iii) Teach your Child to Blow and Suck.

   (iv) Ways to develop Listening Skills.
    (v) Motivation and the Development of Language.
   (vi) Ways to Develop Speech.
  (vii) Ways to Increase Visual and Auditory Memory and Retention.
 (viii) Do's and Don'ts of Speech Development.

Three home visits took place. Parents had an opportunity between visits to read the literature so that its implications for them could be discussed during the next home visit. Home visits were chosen as the means of distributing the literature because they provided families with a means of contact with personnel involved in developing the language programme. Furthermore, there was evidence at this stage that merely posting literature to parents was no guarantee that they would read it thoroughly or indeed apply the teaching suggested (see below p. 98). The value of the home visits at this time was that they provided further information about parents' needs for support services for their child and also about parent attitudes to their participating in a rigorous language training programme.

(e) *Parental Assessment of Children's Language and Parents' Expectations*

This contact took the form of discussion groups with parents. The aim of these discussion groups was to further sensitize parents to the distinctive features of their child's language acquisition. Much of the discussion took the form of examination of parents' knowledge of normal child developmental milestones and of how the pace of child development is slowed by intellectual handicap. Questions were asked of parents about developmental milestones particularly in relation to their own children. Their answers were also an indication as to whether *parents'* expectations for their children were realistic. It seemed reasonable to assume that parental expectations, whether they were high or low, exerted a form of control over their child's learning. For example, such parental assessment and expectations could shape other environmental processes involved in the acquisition of speech and language. In particular, environmental processes such as parent reactions or the establishment of proto-conversational formats could so easily influence a child's learning whatever the stage of development. It is felt that parents' assessment and their expectations are closely associated with the concept of reinforcement for themselves. The implications of what was likely to be effective reinforcement were of singular importance when preparing parents for teaching their intellectually handicapped children.

(f) *Parents' Responses to (i) Task Analysis and (ii) Reinforcer Selection*

After 9 months of contact with parents, a range of specific language tasks and related instructions was presented to parents (see sample of tasks (see Appendix II)). Discussion with parents emphasised the following theme: language is a skill which is hierarchical in nature and, *wherever possible, language tasks will be sequential.* The specific receptive and expressive language tasks were to be seen as external sources of stimulation for each child. The aim of these tasks, therefore, was to activate, maintain, and facilitate the child's language acquisition. The language tasks had to fit the child's level of competence. If the parent could begin teaching at the child's "competence level" then it was reasoned there should be nothing fixed and immutable about the intellectually handicapped child's performance.

Rewards and reinforcer selection

Rewards for their children were discussed with parents in relation to the tasks presented. The aim in these discussions was to take account of individual differences and define rewards accordingly. Since different children like different things, something that is a reinforcer for one child will not necessarily work with all children. The use of edible, social, and manipulatable *rewards* was discussed. It was emphasised that something is called a reinforcement for a child *only when he likes it and will make some effort to get it.* Parents made it clear that in general they favoured social reinforcers. The aim in the discussions was to demonstrate that natural forms of environmental control or reinforcement, especially appropriate social responses such as praise for the child's language production, are generally the most desirable types of reinforcement. However, it was explained to some families that some forms of behaviour that necessarily precede productive language such as fine motor tasks, match-to-sample tasks, and possibly verbal imitation, cannot be easily generated through natural consequences. When natural social consequences fail to maintain behaviour then it was suggested that edible reinforcement such as drinks, crisps, raisins, or possibly ice cream, might be used to "pay" the child to work at a difficult task. Parents were concerned about the misuse of edible reinforcement, feeling that this would lead to the development of quite antisocial habits. Discussions centred around whether there was evidence that edible reinforcement initiated verbal learning and whether the verbal behaviour so acquired would persist so as to make the child intelligible in the natural environment. Emphasis again was placed on the desirability of using social reinforcers, particularly in relation to the long-term aim of generalizing the skill acquired. Edible reinforcers were to be used to develop language behaviours which ultimately would be socially effective. Parents gradually came to accept that when these language behaviours became socially effective then they would not need to be sustained by extrinsic or arbitrary reinforcers such as edibles.

(g) *Selection and Production of the Language Programme*
   The selection of a "suitable" language programme for such a heterogeneous sample posed a problem. Should language development programmes already tried and published be selected or should a programme relevant to parental needs be developed? The decision to write a language teaching programme was taken for a variety of reasons.
   (i) The heterogeneous sample demanded a programme with a wide range of tasks from motor skills acquisition to simple sentence production.
   (ii) Not all parents could have afforded, nor would have purchased, a commercially published programme had it been available, and no cost was incurred by parents in the writing and production of the language manual.
   (iii) Parents had to be involved from the outset if they were to identify with and persist with teaching.
   (iv) In order to measure the effectiveness of the teaching, the language tasks in the manual had to represent measurable criteria (Ch. 4 and Appendix II). Thus, the itemised tasks in the preparatory receptive language and expressive language areas seek to present activities which are *relevant* to the language development of the intellectually handicapped child and to present activities which objectively *measure* the child's language development.

   At the end of Stage I, an itemised language therapy manual entitled *Parents as Language Therapists for Intellectually Handicapped Children* was produced (see Appendix III). This was then distributed to all the families involved in Stage I. The items in the manual represent criterion tasks in a preparatory or motor skills area, receptive language area, and expressive language area. The contents of this manual are presented in Appendix III. These sequential language tasks form the basis for the Parent Training Programme developed in Stage II.

STAGE II — Distinctive Features of the Teaching Programmes
   During this stage the individual child language skills are viewed as the objects of change. As such, Stage II teaching programmes (see above Figure 3.1) had the following characteristics:
   (i) Three different programmes or treatment groups operated: they represented different input from professionals in education, in social work and counselling, and in the paramedical field of speech and occupational therapy.
   (ii) Each distinct programme offered comparable time to parents and their children.
   (iii) Evaluation of language skills acquired by the child as a result of parent and professionals teaching was common to all subjects, no matter what treatment group they belonged to.

Stage II Teaching Programmes
   All of the intellectually handicapped children in this sample were either attending at a local Health and Education Department Therapy Centre or were attending local A.C.T. Schools Authority special schools. It should be emphasised that the treatment programmes (A-C only) represent *additional* professional and parental input via the home and the clinic.

Pre-training for the Teachers, Speech Therapists and Social Workers

All staff involved were professional personnel employed by, or seconded from, the A.C.T. Schools Authority and the Capital Territory Health Commission. Pre-training for these professionals took the form of:

(a) reading the Language Therapy Manual and discussing its contents with the research staff. In these discussions, the *sequential* and itemised nature of the language programme was stressed as was the close relationship between language tasks and the criterion language measures (see Appendices Ib and Ic);

(b) learning about the criterion language profile at O_2 (Figure 3.1 and Appendix V) and the form of daily and weekly assessment of children on the prescribed language tasks (see below Chapter 7);

(c) testing the children by teachers and psychologists who were familiar to each child: the children were tested on the preparatory receptive and expressive tasks in the manual (see Appendix II). Each child's scores on all the tasks were recorded and a language profile based on the criterion measures was achieved (see Ch. 4, p. 70 and Appendix V).

The performance charts indicate where criterion was not achieved (see sample language profile chart, Appendix V and Case Studies, Chapter 7). This determines which language tasks parents should begin teaching. After consultation with the speech therapists and teachers, parents were informed which tasks had been selected for teaching. Thereafter, direct daily assessment by parents of their child's language behaviour took place. These assessments were brought by parents to group training sessions. Weekly assessment also took place in local special schools, at health centres or the therapy centre by trained independent observers. This weekly assessment represents the language criterion achieved each week for each child. The characteristics of these criterion language measures are that as near as possible they are precisely defined, are easily identifiable and involve assessment by parents and/or professionals of directly observable actions. Weekly assessment took place over 30 weeks during Stage II. Receptive and expressive language tasks were changed as soon as criterion scores were recorded (see below Chapter 7). It should be emphasised that the teachers, speech therapists, psychologists and social workers involved in the programme were most experienced in working with these children. Each treatment programme therefore is a reflection of their experience. In view of this professional experience no more *pre-training* took place other than that which has been indicated.

The comparative study of treatment programmes rests on the basis that:

(i) the treatments were different for all groups from O_2 to O_4 (see Figure 3.1) and

(ii) the *sequence* of treatment was different from O_2 to O_5 or O_2 to O_6 (see Figure 3.1).

The sequence of treatment may be best understood by careful examination of Figure 3.1. It needs to be emphasised that while three groups received the structured target teaching programme, groups B and C only received that intervention after either six months of social work/supportive counselling or six months of speech therapy.

Distinctive Features of Group A. Target Tearching $O_2 — O_5$: Figure 3.1

This particular programme is concerned with instructing parents in the use of structured behaviour modification techniques for teaching their own children. The distinctive features of this programme are:

(a) Language tasks for teaching were selected for each child according to the results achieved on the language profiles at O_2 (see Figure 3.1, and Appendices I, II and III and sample language profile Appendix V). To begin with, the tasks chosen were those that a child could possibly *just attain and then, with support, practice and maintain.*

(b) Group A parents entered into an agreement/contract that they would receive individual language target teaching with their children on condition that they participated in the behaviour modification group training sessions. No such contract was formed with any other treatment group.

(c) Parents had a minimum of 16 x 2½ hour *group* training sessions during the period O_2 to O_5 (see Fig. 3.1). Group training took the form of demonstrations, discussion groups and viewing of video films of parent and professional teaching. No group training took place during school holiday periods. The principles of the behaviour modification techniques outlined in group training sessions were as follows:

  (i)   Select the language targets (preparatory and/or receptive language tasks) to be taught.

 (ii)   Shape or physically help the child to imitate a large class of general responses (generally gross motor responses) by the teacher/therapist. Aim to develop this class of responses to the point where selective reinforcement could be attempted. This was introduced early to demonstrate reinforcement principles with responses each child was possibly already capable of. Relate this teaching to the section on imitation in the language manual (see Appendix II and Chapter 7).

(iii)   Define and demonstrate the technique of successive approximation; that is, help the child to imitate more specific responses demonstrated by the teacher/therapist by concurrently reinforcing the "prompted" imitated responses. Generally encourage the use of social reinforcers and emphasise the personal characteristics of the teacher/ therapist and parent as a human reinforcer.

(iv)   Slowly remove the physical prompts step by step and reinforce closer and closer approximations to the modelled target response.

 (v)   When the modelled target response has been achieved (e.g. pointing to three named objects) then *rehearse* the procedure until the defined criterion for each task could be repeated whenever required.

(vi)   Apply the same procedures (i) to (v) above to establish vocal imitations (expressive language tasks). Essentially, demonstrate that training of vocal responses consists of providing closer and closer matches to responses demonstrated by the teacher/ therapist or parent. Emphasise that any expressive language or vocal imitation training be preceded by training receptive language tasks, most of which require motor responses. The expressive language tasks in the language manual (see Appendix II) have been so arranged that *vocal* training necessitates linking the required receptive language and motor response to associated expressive responses.

(d) In addition to the group training sessions (referred to in (c) (i) — (vi) above), children accompanied by their parents received a one-half-hour-per-week individual behaviour modification/language-training session according to the specified tasks. A minimum of 25 one-half-hour sessions with the teacher/therapist was achieved for each child in group A. The teacher/therapist carried out the language training in the first two months and then parents were gradually encouraged to take over. Random selections of training sessions were videotaped for demonstration in group training sessions.*

Distinctive Features of Group B. Social Work/Supportive Counselling Programme. 0_2—0_4: Figure 3.1

    This programme is concerned with giving social work services and supportive counselling to the families.^ø This *six month* programme (see Figure 3.1) represents the input according to professional role of the social worker/supportive counsellor (Bayley 1973; Hewett 1970; Schild 1971). The distinctive features of this programme were:

(a) Language tasks for teaching were selected for each child according to the results achieved on the language profiles at 0_2 (see Figure 3.1 and Appendices I, II, III and IV and sample language profile Appendix VI). To begin with, the tasks chosen were those that a child could possibly just attain and then maintain.

(b) There was no agreement/contract about the relationship between individual home visits and group discussion sessions.

---

* Videotapes used: High Density J Standard Sony AV 34/20: Portapack.

ø There is no simple relationship between such essentially social transactions and outcome. Characterisation of this programme from the social worker/supportive counsellor's point of view is what is "defined" below in (c) (i) — (viii).

(c) Parents received a maximum of ten, minimum of six social worker/supportive-counsellor group training sessions of three hours' duration during the period O_2 to O_4. This is considered comparable with the contact time received by Group A and Group C. The principles and content of these group meetings were as follows:
  (i) Listen to and record parents' point of view about their child's development;
  (ii) Counsel parents where necessary about their child's future development;
  (iii) Listen to and record parents' points of view about their expectations from the programme;
  (iv) Listen to and counsel parents about their daily problems of coping with an intellectually handicapped child;
  (v) Listen to and counsel parents about their opportunities for teaching their child on a daily bais;
  (vi) Listen to and record parents' points of view about the social worker/supportive counsellor's role;
  (vii) Social workers/supportive counsellors enlarge parents' understanding of the nature and prognosis of intellectual handicap;
  (viii) Social workers/supportive counsellors help parents to use the language manual.
(d) Individual home visits once every two weeks to provide *individual* contact and help with the language programme. Where necessary, social workers liaised with other agencies such as special schools and counselling services in the Capital Territory Health Commission.

Distinctive Features of Group B. Target Teaching O_4—O_5: Figure 3.1
  The Target Teaching programme as outlined for Group A above was given to group B for the final three months of Stage II. Six 2½ hour group-training sessions were held during the three months, and the families also received ten individual one-half-hour target-teaching sessions with the teacher/therapist comparable with those outline for the Target Teaching Group A (see above).

Distinctive Features of Group C. Speech Therapy Programme O_2—O_4: Figure 3.1
  This programme was concerned with instructing parents in the use of language stimulation principles analogous to those used in speech therapy (Wood 1964). The distinctive features outlined by the speech therapists were:
(a) Parents and speech therapists were *advised* of the language levels selected for each child according to the results achieved on the language profiles at O_2 (see Figure 3.1 and Appendices II and III and sample language profile Appendix V). However, the speech therapists and parents were to select language related activities based on what *they* felt the child could do and was interested in.
(b) Group C parents had no agreement/contract with regard to the provision of individual speech therapy for their children. Individual speech therapy sessions based on ten one-half-hour appointments was the minimum number required for children's data to be included for analysis O_2—O_4.
(c) Parents had a minimum of ten speech therapy/*group*-discussion sessions in small groups during the three month period (O_2—O_4). This is comparable with the contact time received by Group A and Group B. The principles and content of these speech therapy/*discussion* groups were as follows:
  (i) Reference was made to the *sequential* items in the language manual (see Appendices II and III).
  (ii) The *role* of the child was stressed. His *interests* were emphasised in contrast to the defined targets outlined for Group A. For example, "Allow the child to demonstrate what he can do and what he has been successful at doing" and "Take your language cues from the child" were adhered to principles of the speech therapy approach.
  (iii) Speech therapy began with activities which approximated to the level at which the child was operating or, indeed, somewhat below it. Parents were requested to select individual teaching materials which were appropriate to the child's mental age and

encouraged to allow the child to select and play with specific toys and, furthermore, to guide and stimulate his playing with these toys.
   (iv) Therapy was made cohesive by planning activities which could be continued at home by the child's parents. The parents were guided in the use and development of speech therapy at home, and encouraged to duplicate equipment/materials used in therapy sessions. Emphasis was given to facilitating parent-child interaction.
   (v) The importance of the receptive (input) language area was stressed, particularly in relation to child play. This was discussed in the light of the definitions of the auditory and visual modalities as set out in the manual (see Appendix III). At all times help the child to understand the *input* of language without any *explicit* attempt to produce a verbal response.
(d) Children accompanied by their parents received a minimum of ten, one-half-hour speech therapy sessions each week. The speech therapist carried out the speech therapy in the first two months and then parents were gradually encouraged to take over. Random selections of training sessions were videotaped for demonstration in group training sessions.*
(e) Parents were encouraged to carry out speech therapy in the home on a *daily basis* according to the principles outlined above (c. i — v). Parents were encouraged to maintain daily records, to undertake audio recordings and to bring these to group training sessions.

Distinctive Features of Group C. Target Teaching 0_4 to 0_5: Figure 3.1
   The Target Teaching programme as outlined for Group A above was given to Group C for the final three months of Stage II. Six 2½ hour group training sessions were held during the three months and the families also received ten individual one-half-hour target teaching sessions with the teacher/therapist comparable with those outlined for the Target Teaching Group A.

Distinctive Features of Group D. Language Programme Only 0_2—0_5: Figure 3.1
   The families in this group were given the language manual *Parents as Language Therapists for Intellectually Handicapped Children* (see Appendix III). They were advised as to the language level selected for their child according to the language profiles at 0_2 (see Figure 3.1, and Appendices II and sample language profile Appendix VI). Thereafter, no more contact took place between these families and members of the research team until the commencement of Stage III one year later.

STAGE III — Distinctive Features of the Treatment Programme for one year 0_5 to 0_6: Figure 3.1
   This programme is common to *all* subjects. It consisted of:
   (i) Informing schools and parents of the availability of language therapy services and where these could be obtained. Once this advice had been given no further initiative was taken by the research team other than to facilitate contact with speech therapy services where necessary.
   (ii) Parents taking the initiative to contact the speech/language therapist to arrange for appointments. Only parents who kept appointments or made contact with the speech therapists are included in this study.
   (iii) Appointments took place in the parent's homes, at Health Centres, or in A.C.T. Schools Authority Special Schools.
   (iv) Consultation, advice and demonstration of language therapy techniques was the form of therapy offered. The importance of the parents' role in developing the child's language skills was emphasised and encouraged.
   (v) Speech therapists undertook to examine and provide therapy where individual difficulties were pointed out by parents.
   (vi) Speech/language therapists kept records of all appointments made prior to the terminal evaluation at 0_6 (see Figure 3.1).

* Videotapes used: High Density J Standard Sony AV 34/20: Portapack.

Chapter Four

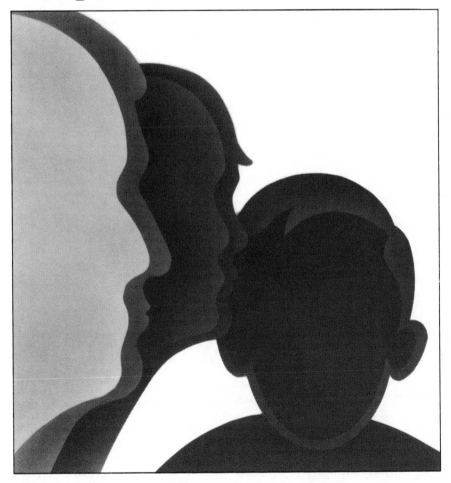

Research Design and Procedures

ASSESSMENT PROCEDURES

(i) The one hundred and two children in this study (see above Ch. 1 p. 8) were those who were taught and assessed throughout the programme 0_1 to 0_6 inclusive. All of these children completed the Reynell Developmental Language Scales Verbal Comprehension Test (which is known hereafter as the Reynell Receptive Language Test (RRLA) and the Reynell Expressive Language Test (RELA) (Reynell 1969b) at the commencement of the programme, at observation point 0_1 and at the following post-test observation points 0_2 to 0_6 inclusive.

(ii) Eighty-seven children above a chronological age of 2½ years at the commencement of the programme at 0_1 were assessed on the Stanford Binet IQ test (Form LM) and of these, sixty-six children received the post-test at the termination of the programme at 0_6 (see above Ch. 1, p. 10 and Fig. 3.1, Ch. 3). This 24 per cent fallout is accounted for by children whose families left the A.C.T., or who withdrew from the programme, or who were not available for the post-test at observation point 0_6.

(iii) Parents of one hundred and one children completed Strom's Parent as a Teacher (PAAT) attitude inventory (Strom and Slaughter 1976) at observation point 0_2 by means of individual interviews. One family did not complete the PAAT questionnaire form though their child completed all other language tests in the programme (see (i) above) — hence the 101 families. The PAAT was used in order to both counsel parents about their attitude to teaching their children and to evaluate the relationship between parents' expressed attitudes and their children's measured language development.

(iv) All one hundred and two children were also tested on the itemised language profile at 0_2 (see Appendix V) and undertook the appropriate weekly criterion reference language measures of the particular receptive and expressive language tasks being taught by their parents. Thirty weekly probes of criterion receptive and expressive language measures were recorded independently by teachers or therapists, not involved in the clinic teaching. All one hundred and two children received these probes during the period 0_2 to 0_5 (See Fig. 3.1). Daily measures over the period 0_2 to 0_5 took place for a random sample (see below Ch. 7).

DISTRIBUTION OF FAMILIES INTO TREATMENT GROUPS

At observation point 0_2 the one hundred and two children in the sample were listed in rank order according to their combined mean observed RRLA and RELA scores at 0_1. (See Table 4.1). This stratified sample took the following form:

(a) Children with a combined receptive and expressive language mean score of 18 months or less were designated as Level 1.

(b) Children with a combined receptive and expressive language mean score of above 18 months but not more than 36 months were designated as Level 2.

(c) Children with a combined receptive and expressive language mean score above 36 months were designated as Level 3.

Stratified random sampling was used to obtain a representative sample for each treatment group at the beginning of Stage II at observation point 0_2. The number of children per language level in each experimental group at 0_2 is set out in Table 4.1. These three language age levels were also used as a basis for demonstrating and explaining to parents the sequential stage of language development (see above Ch. 3 and below Ch. 7).

TABLE 4.1

Number of Children per Language Level at O_2

in each Experimental Treatment Group

	Group A	Group B	Group C	Group D
Level 1	11	12	13	13
Level 2	9	8	7	10
Level 3	5	4	5	5

MODIFICATIONS TO THE ORIGINAL STRATIFIED RANDOM DISTRIBUTION

In view of the nature of parents' involvement and of the experimental Target Teaching programme, two modifications to the original stratified distrubition were made.

(i) If parents strongly objected to their child being placed in the Language programme Only Group D this had to be taken into account. Therefore, those twenty-eight children in the Language Programme only Group D (see Tables 4.1 and 4.2) are those whose parents did not object to this placement. Reference is made to this sampling bias in the results in Ch. 5. However, in the sample of 102 families, only two of them from the original distribution in Group D were placed in other treatment groups.

(ii) Parents of children placed in the Target Teaching Group A had to accept the contract arrangements of the group or withdraw from the group (see above Ch. 3 p. 58). The contract was quite specific. Parents would only receive individual, weekly, target teaching training with their child, if they agreed to attend, regular, weekly, parent group training sessions in operant target teaching techniques. Parents of younger children were more willing to accept this contract.

Therefore, those families originally placed in Group A but unable to participate in the weekly training programme were then placed in Groups B, C and D. As a result, the mean chronological age for Group A of 5 years 2 months (see Table 4.3) was seven months or more younger than the mean ages for the other treatment groups.

INSTRUMENTATION

(i) *The Reynell Developmental Language Scales*

The Reynell Development Language Scales (Reynell 1969b) were used to assess the children's receptive and expressive language performance. The Scales have a developmental orientation. They provide language age measures in the areas of receptive language or verbal comprehension and expressive language. Although language development is conveniently assessed by the yardstick of spoken utterances it is also equally important to know how far the intellectually handicapped understand what is said. Mittler (1974) is quite explicit that Reynell's receptive and expressive language tests are particularly useful in the assessment of the language of the handicapped. In contrast with Piaget's position (Piaget 1926) Reynell believes that "language is the vehicle for thought" (Reynell 1969b, p. 13). For example, in her description of the measures of a child's verbal comprehension Reynell writes:

> The order of this scale follows the development of verbal comprehension from the earliest stage of selective recognition of certain word patterns on an affective level, through gradually increasing complexity of interpretation of different parts of speech, to the stage at which verbal interpretation extends to situations beyond the here and now, and language becomes a true vehicle of thought. After this point, verbal comprehension becomes linked to increasingly complex intellectual processes, and to increasing vocabulary knowledge, merging into other intellectual processes to such an extent that it can no longer be assessed as a relatively separate function. For this reason the ceiling is set developmentally. The process of verbal comprehension develops rapidly from the age of about 7 months up to 5 or 6 years, after which time it becomes increasingly a 'tool' process for higher intellectual functions . . . (Reynell 1969b, p. 10).

In this description can be observed the likely overlap between verbal comprehension, or receptive language skills and measures of concept attainment related to "knowledge of vocabulary, comprehension and development of memory". Reynell's verbal comprehension or receptive language scales (RRLA) deal with such matters as: the child's first understanding of names of familiar objects, the ability to relate concepts, the ability to understand and carry out simple instructions, and the ability to comprehend the relationship between nouns, verbs and other parts of speech in one sentence. It is these skills which, for Reynell, are indicative of receptive language and which can be "assessed as a separate function".

There are two parallel comprehension or receptive language scales. Scale 'A' used in this research is dependent on some hand function (rather than just the use of eye-pointing), but does not need speech. The aim of the receptive language test is to give a quantitative estimate of a child's level of comprehension relative to norms for his or her age, and to elucidate in a qualitative way (see Ch. 5) any aspect or stage of comprehension which may be particularly difficult for the intellectually handicapped.

Reynell's verbal language input-output sequence (Reynell 1969a) is reproduced in diagram form in Fig. 4.1 p. 68.

TABLE 4.2

Number and Distribution of Children in Treatment Groups

Etiology	Group A		Group B		Group C		Group D	
	Boys	Girls	Boys	Girls	Boys	Girls	Boys	Girls
Down's Syndrome	7	10	8	5	7	4	9	7
Brain Damaged	2	3	4	2	-	1	1	3
Epilepsy	-	-	1	-	2	1	-	1
Hydrocephaly	-	-	1	-	-	-	-	-
Microcephaly	2	1	-	1	2	1	1	1
Genetic Disorder	-	-	1	-	3	-	-	-
Mentally Handicapped[6]	-	-	1	-	3	1	3	2
TOTAL	11	14	16	8	17	8	14	14
Group Total	N = 25		N = 24		N = 25		N = 28	

TABLE 4.3

Mean Chronological Ages of Children in Months in Treatment Groups

Etiology	Group A		Group B		Group C		Group D	
	Boys	Girls	Boys	Girls	Boys	Girls	Boys	Girls
Down's Syndrome	50	62	64	63	72	52	76	51
Brain Damaged	102	72	81	78	-	20	118	55
Epilepsy	-	-	88	-	50	97	-	70
Hydrocephaly	-	-	54	-	-	-	-	-
Microcephaly	65	40	-	96	50	55	43	45
Genetic Disorder	-	-	46	-	73	-	-	-
Mentally Handicapped∅	-	-	108	-	109	114	92	79
TOTAL MEAN	62	63	71	71	74	62	80	58
GROUP MEAN	62		71		70		69	

∅ Mental Handicap: Children whose intellectual handicap is due to no known organic origin.

Fig. 4.1

VERBAL LANGUAGE INPUT-OUTPUT SEQUENCE

Hearing for Speech → Receptive Language → Central Organisation → Expressive Language → Speech Mechanism

This diagram demonstrates the relationship between a child's verbal comprehension or receptive language skills and the child's speech or expressive language. The Reynell expressive language scale has three sections. Section 1 "taps the very earliest stages of pre-language from the earliest vocalisations to the use of complex sentences with subordinate clauses". In Section 2 the vocabulary required increases in difficulty . . . "and yet the words are chosen so that they are within the experience of even the most housebound handicapped child" (Reynell 1969b Ch. 4, p. 14). Section 3 is in Reynell's terms concerned with the assessment of the more creative uses of language. As such, success in this section identifies those children who are "able to verbalise connected thoughts which is the creative use of language".

The Reynell Developmental Language test material consists of every day objects such as: cup, spoon, brush, sock, and toys such as: cars, dolls, and farm animals. These objects have been found to be familiar to most intellectually handicapped children. The vocabulary used in both the receptive and expressive language tests is kept simple throughout. Increasing difficulty is related to sentence length and ideational content.

(ii) *The Revised Stanford Binet IQ Test (Form LM).*

The revised Stanford Binet (Form LM) was the instrument used to assess the children's IQ scores (see Ch. 1 p. 10 and Table 1.4). It is an age scale which makes use of age standards of performance. The Stanford Binet sets out to measure intelligence regarded as "general mental adaptability" (Terman and Merrill 1960, Ch. 3, p. 62).

Baroff (1974) stated that from the point of view of early childhood until adolescence the Stanford Binet is the single most useful intelligence test for use with children who are suspected of retardation (Baroff 1974, p. 137).

However, it should be noted, that the heavier weighting given to verbal items at successfully higher levels on the Stanford Binet, is considered, to be a reason for the slight lowering of IQ scores as children get older (MacCubrey 1971).

The factors which account for a child's achievement in intelligence tests according to Hofstaetter (1954) are: (i) sensorimotor alertness; (ii) persistence; and (iii) manipulation of symbols. In his factor analyses of the inter-age correlations of Bayley's 18 year growth study Hofstaetter demonstrated that *alertness* accounts for the variance of mental age scores for the first two years. The majority of the children in this "Parents as Language Therapists" study come within this *mental age group*. Hofstaetter considers that between two and four years of age the second factor *persistence* is operative and after four years of age the skill *manipulation of symbols* is to the fore. These skills are involved in a child "transforming reality, conferring personal meaning and representing what is perceived". Prominent among sub-test items that appear in the revised Stanford Binet are vocabulary, comprehension, concepts such as opposites, similarities and differences, verbal and pictorial completions, copying and drawing designs, and memory for common objects.

It is evident that Stanford Binet scores typically correlate better with tests requiring a high degree of verbal skill, indicating that the Stanford Binet is highly saturated with these skills, (Kennedy, Van de Reit and White 1963; McCubrey 1971). However, satisfactory levels of correlation with other measures of intelligence have been reported (Himelstein 1966). For example, a correlation of 0.74 between the Stanford Binet (Form LM) and the Wechsler Intelligence Scale for Children was reported by Estes, Curtin, DeBurger and Deny (1961). The use of the Stanford Binet in this research, was accepted by both parents and the different groups of professionals involved, as a means of assessing the children's general mental adaptability.

(iii) *Strom's Parent as a Teacher (PAAT) attitude inventory*

The Parent as a Teacher Inventory (PAAT) (Strom & Slaughter 1976) is a composite attitude scale in which individual parents describe feelings about various aspects of the parent-child interactive system. In responding to the PAAT (see Appendix VII) parents of the intellectually handicapped were able to demonstrate their standards for assessing the importance of various aspects of child behaviour. This was the first time that this instrument has been used in which the focus has been on parents' attitudes to their intellectually handicapped children. An aim in using the PAAT was to examine the assumption that many of the attitudes about appropriate parental responses to teaching normal children would be relevant for effective parent-training for this group.

The rationale for using such an instrument in the "Parents as Language Therapists" programme was that (a) individual parent's emotional and behavioural responses to his or her child are related to value loaded expectations about his or her child's retardation and level of skills, (b) individual parent's current parenting experiences are likely to affect their willingness to teach and persist with teaching their children and (c) individual parents have definite beliefs regarding child behaviour and this affects their attitudes to different teaching programmes.

The PAAT provided the method of examining these factors from an individual parent's point of view. The PAAT provided the means of examining the relationship between parent and child development and provided a guide for feedback to individual parents. This feedback was also a guide to programme planning for language teaching, both in the clinic setting and in the children's homes.

The instrument was first developed for measuring child-rearing expectations related to the intellectual and creative development of preschool and kindergarten children of normal or above average intelligence. A complete description of the measure, including reliability and validity studies, has been reported (Strom and Johnson, 1978; Strom and Slaughter, 1978) and adapted use of this instrument with single parent Australian families has also been demonstrated and reported (Constable et al 1979; Drake-Brockman 1979).

The items contained in the PAAT (See Appendix VII) include a wide variety of statements about what parents want or expect of their child, how they respond to specific aspects of their interaction with their child and what actions parents take in response to specific child behaviour. PAAT responses were grouped into subsets of 10 items each related to five areas of parent curriculum:

1. Creativity subset — parental acceptance of creative functioning in their intellectually handicapped child and desire to encourage or suppress its development.
2. Frustration subset — parent childrearing frustration and locus of the frustration.
3. Control subset — parent feelings about control and the extent to which parental control of their intellectually handicapped child's behaviour was deemed necessary.
4. Play subset — parental understanding of play and its influence on their intellectually handicapped child's development.
5. Teaching-Learning subset — parental perception of their own ability to facilitate the teaching-learning process for their intellectually handicapped child.

PAAT directions told the respondents that they would read statements on feelings about their children and assured them that the inventory was not a test but rather a means to express their own feelings (see Appendix VII). They were asked to circle only one answer per item. Each PAAT item has four possible answers: Strong Yes, Yes, No, Strong No. The answers always appeared in the same order. If they had no doubt about a statement, parents were directed to circle Strong Yes or Strong No. Otherwise, they were asked to circle Yes or No, indicating the direction of their feelings concerning each of the 50 statements. There was no time limit.

Scoring the inventory calls for assigning a numerical value of 4, 3, 2 or 1 to each of the 50 responses. The most desired responses (according to Strom and Slaughter, 1978) based upon child development research were valued 4, with diminishing values assigned to other responses on the basis of their distance from the most desirable. Scoring may begin from left to right. For example, the most desirable answer for item 29 was Strong Yes, while the most desirable response for item 39 was Strong No. Both responses would be valued 4.

		Strong Yes	Yes	No	Strong No
29.	My child learns new words when we play.	4	3	2	1
39.	It is difficult for me to stay interested when playing with my child.	1	2	3	4

Respondents who circled other answers would receive the lower values as shown. The PAAT Inventory was constructed with 27 items having Strong No as the desired response.

After values were assigned to each response, subtotals were derived for parents' attitude to creativity, frustration, control, play, and the teaching learning process (see below Ch. 6). The total score was then obtained by summing all five subtotals (see below Ch. 6). Whenever an item was thought to be inapplicable to parents with intellectually handicapped children, it was discussed by the interviewer and parent and a qualitative assessment, as well as a numerical value was obtained.

(iv) *Criterion Reference Language Measures for Receptive and Expressive Language Skills*
At the end of Stage 1 (see Ch. 3 Fig 3.1 and Appendix II) an itemised language teaching manual was produced. The receptive and expressive language items in this manual provided parents and professionals with language tasks and related measurements. These measurements of children's receptive and expressive language skills were absolute indices. They were designed to indicate which receptive or expressive language tasks a child had or had not learned from a given instructional segment (see below Ch. 7).

70

These language measurements (see Appendix II and below Ch. 7) were absolute in that they were interpretable solely vis-a-vis a fixed performance standard or criterion and need not be interpreted relative to other language measurements. The receptive and expressive language measures in the case studies reported in Ch. 7 indicate what a child had or had not learned. What any one child had learned was indicated by his/her successful completion of particular language tasks, which in turn may be compared to the total range of language tasks in the language manual that any child in this programme could possibly learn.

These language measurements (see Appendix II), are considered to be representative of the skills taught. Parents in each group had copies of the language manual (see Ch. 3, p. 57) and the language tasks that were taught came from the language manual.

Single case experimental designs are used increasingly in clinical research. Their unique contribution in this study is that they can experimentally evaluate the home base language teaching intervention for the individual child. The single case experimental teaching of receptive and expressive language reported in Chapter 7 is based on careful observation of the children's receptive and expressive language behaviour during a baseline phase at observation point O_2 (see above p. 61). The data collected during the baseline phase described the level of each child's receptive and expressive language performance (see Appendix V) and hence provided information about the extent of each child's language difficulties. Secondly, the criterion language profile data collected at observation point O_2 served as a basis for predicting the children's level of performance for the immediate future if specific teaching was not provided.

Data collected during the specific teaching phase stage II, (see also Ch. 7) provided evidence of the children's new levels of performance in receptive and expressive language. This was used in discussion with parents to predict how the children's language skills might develop in the immediate future, if the teaching was continued.

Two designs are most commonly used in single case experimentation. These designs are the A B A B or reversal design and the multiple baseline design. The A B A B design evaluates an intervention by alternating the baseline condition (A phase) when no treatment is in effect with the intervention (B phase). However, once the specific teaching began after O_2 (see Fig 3.1 p. 54 and below Tables 4.4 and 4.5) then the teaching continued until O_5 at the end of Stage II (see Fig. 3.1, p. 54). Therefore a multiple baseline design as recommended by Baer, Wolf and Risley (1965) was used. Although there are different versions of the multiple baseline design (Kazdin 1978), the design used here was one in which receptive and expressive language data were collected on a daily and weekly basis. The specific experimental teaching on particular receptive or expressive language tasks ceased once criterion on that task had been achieved.

The therapeutic criterion for evaluation of these single case studies was the value, or importance, of the changes in children's receptive and expressive language skills. This criterion referred to whether the extent of behaviour change achieved during treatment enhanced the children's functioning in everyday situations. Implicit in this criterion was that the receptive or expressive language tasks selected for teaching were of clinical and social importance. This criterion is referred to in Chapter 7.

Five case studies encompassing a range of receptive and expressive language tasks are presented. These case studies cover the range of receptive and expressive language tasks that appear in the language manual (see Chapter 3, p. 57 and Appendix III). They are also cases in which both daily and weekly receptive and expressive language scores were reliably collected. The detailed case studies presented in Chapter 7, cover the following receptive and expressive language tasks:

  (i) Responding correctly to ten simple commands.
 (ii) Naming ten everyday objects.
(iii) Responding correctly to prepositional requests.
 (iv) Vocalising three imitative speech sounds.
  (v) Identifying pictures from general descriptions.
 (vi) Describing pictures by using noun phrases.

RESEARCH QUESTIONS

Chapter 1 and Chapter 3 outline the problems, aims, and teaching included in this "Parents as Language Therapists Programme". The chief research questions being asked were:

(i) Which teaching methods were most likely to maximise the receptive and expressive language development of intellectually handicapped children and for how long should these teaching programmes be applied?

(ii) Did a child's sex or etiology affect the development of receptive and expressive language skills?

(iii) Did a child's stage or level of language development affect the success of different teaching programmes?

(iv) To what extent were an intellectually handicapped child's IQ scores reliable and what was the relationship between IQ scores and language age scores?

(v) What was the nature of the relationship between the child-rearing expectations of parents of intellectually handicapped children and parents' ability to teach their children language skills?

(vi) To what extent can individual case studies demonstrate the way in which children respond, or fail to respond to different treatments and different language tasks?

STATISTICAL ANALYSIS

(i) To adjust for initial differences between treatment groups a multivariate analysis of covariance (MANCOVA) was used (Bock 1975). In this analysis the Reynell Receptive Language Age (RRLA) scores or the Reynell Expressive Language Age (RELA) scores at observation points O_1 and O_2 (see Fig. 3.1 p. 54) were used as covariates. Similarly, to adjust for initial differences within treatment groups, due for example to quite different stages of language development at the commencement of the programme, then MANCOVA was also used.

The multivariate analysis of covariance (MANCOVA) was used because it was logical to consider controlling the RRLA or the RELA scores experimentally by equalising the treatment groups or the language levels groups within treatment groups on the basis of the RRLA or RELA variables. This equalising was carried out statistically through the multivariate analysis of covariance (MANCOVA) where it effected adjustments on the various post-test RRLA or RELA scores.

The multivariate analysis of covariance is an adjunct to the multivariate analysis of variance. It is in effect a multivariate analysis of variance (MANOVA) of the adjusted RRLA or RELA scores.

(ii) Multivariate analysis of variance (MANOVA) of the repeated RRLA or RELA scores at observation points O_1, O_2, O_3, O_4, O_5, and O_6 or at observation points O_3, O_4, O_5 and O_6 was used when the influence on the children's language development of factors such as sex and etiology were being examined. Similarly MANOVA of the RRLA or RELA scores at observation points O_1 to O_6 or at observation points O_3 to O_6 was used to demonstrate whether the difference between children's different language levels within treatment groups was statistically significant.

The "exclusive" multivariate approach (Bock 1975 p. 426) is represented by the step-down F tests in which the dependent variables Reynell Receptive Language Age (RRLA) scores were successively shifted to the role of independent variables. This means that the less informative or redundant variables (RRLA at observation points O_1 to O_6 or RELA at observation points O_1 and O_2 (see Fig. 3.1 p. 54) were used as covariates. Similarly, to adjust for initial differences within treatment groups, due for example to quite different

(iii) To examine the relationship between Stanford Binet IQ observed scores at the commencement and termination of the programme and the relationship between Stanford

Binet IQ scores and the Reynell Receptive (RRLA) or Expressive Language (RELA) observed scores, the Pearson product-moment correlation coefficient (r) indicated the way in which the variables referred to above related to each other.

(iv) Testing for significance between different parent group scores on the PAAT involved the use of Cochran and Cox's formula for testing the significance of the computed t when variances differ, as shown by an F test (Cochran 1963, Cochran and Cox 1957).

RESEARCH DESIGN

The research design adopted (see Fig. 3.1) can also be characterised as in Table 4.4.

TABLE 4.4

Diagrammatic Representation of Research
Design Procedures

Gp	Pt	T	R	Pt	T	Po	T	Po	T	Po	T	Po
A	0_1	X_1	R	0_2	X_2	0_3	X_2	0_4	X_2	0_5	X_6	0_6
B	0_1	X_1	R	0_2	X_3	0_3	X_3	0_4	X_2	0_5	X_6	0_6
C	0_1	X_1	R	0_2	X_4	0_3	X_4	0_4	X_2	0_5	X_6	0_6
D	0_1	X_1	R	0_2	X_5	0_3	X_5	0_4	X_5	0_5	X_6	0_6

R = Stratified Random Distribution. T = Treatment X_1, X_2, X_3, X_4, X_5 or X_6

Pt (Pre-test) 0_1, 0_2 before experimental treatments X_2 to X_5

Po = Post-test, 0_3, 0_4, 0_5, and 0_6

DESIGN PROCEDURE

(i) The subjects were pretested on the receptive and expressive language dependent variables: Reynell Developmental Language Scale (Reynell, 1969b) and on the Stanford Binet (Form LM) Intelligence Scale (Terman and Merrill, 1961).

(ii) All subjects were exposed for one year to the common intervention (independent variable) X_1 (see above Ch. 3 and Figure 3.1).

(iii) The subjects were assigned to treatment groups by stratified random distribution (see above p. 65). The treatments Target Teaching X_2, Social Work/Supportive Counselling X_3, Speech Therapy X_4, and the Language Programme only X_5 were also assigned to groups by random methods.

(iv) The subjects were pre-tested at observation points 0_2, (Fig. 3.1) on the dependent variables: Reynell Receptive Language Scale (RRLA) and Expressive Language Scale (RELA) (Reynell, 1969b).

(v) The subjects were tested on Preparatory, Receptive and Expressive tasks independently, as outlined in the Language Criterion Check List (see Appendix II). Weekly Criterion measures of each child's Preparatory, Receptive and Expressive Language skills followed for the next 30 weeks (Stage II, see above p. 70 and Figure 3.1 p. 54).

73

(vi) The subjects were pre-tested at observation point O_2 (see above Figure 3.1 and p. 69) on the Parent as a Teacher Attitude Inventory (PAAT) (Strom, 1976).

(vii) The experimental group A, and Groups, B, C and D (see above Ch. 3) were exposed to the respective treatments; X_2 Target Teaching, X_3 Social Work/Supportive Counselling, and X_4 Speech Therapy or X_5 Language Programme only, for three months (also see above Fig. 3.1).

(viii) At the end of the first twelve weeks of intervention all subjects were post-tested at observation point O_3 on the dependent variables RRLA and RELA as in (iv) above.

(ix) The experimental group A, and Groups B, C and D were further exposed to the respective treatments X_2, X_3, X_4 and X_5 for a further 12 weeks.

(x) At the end of this second twelve week period of treatment (from O_3 to O_4, see above Fig. 3.1) all subjects were post-tested at observation point O_4 on the dependent variables RRLA and RELA as for (iv) and (viii) above.

(xi) The experimental groups A, B and C were all exposed to common treatment Target Teaching X_2 for twelve weeks. Group D still received no specific additional intervention (also see above Figure 3.1).

(xii) At the end of this final twelve week period (see above Figure 3.1) all subjects were post-tested at observation point O_5 on the dependent variables RRLA and RELA as for (iv), (viii) and (x) above.

(xiii) All subjects were also post-tested on the Parent As A Teacher Attitude Inventory (PAAT) as in (vi) above.

(xiv) All subjects in Groups A, B, C and D were provided with the common Speech Therapy Services X_6 for one year (Stage III Figure 3.1).

(xv) All subjects were post-tested at observation point O_6 on the dependent variables RRLA and RELA as outlined in (iv), (viii), (x) and (xii) above. At observation point O_6 (see Figure 3.1) this also included the Stanford Binet (Form LM) Intelligence Scale as for (i) above.

ANALYSIS PROCEDURE

(i) The differences between the mean scores on each dependent variable for each group separately and for each subgroup were computed according to the hypotheses presented.

(ii) The differences among the groups and between the groups were compared to determine whether the application X_2 Target Teaching or X_3 Social Work/Supportive Counselling or X_4 Speech Therapy or X_5 Language Programme only was associated with a change in the experimental Group A compared to Groups B, C or D.

(iii) The difference between measures for boys and girls or etiology groups were compared to determine the relationship of these factors to children's receptive and expressive language development.

(iv) The relationship of children's IQ scores at the commencement and termination of the programme (O_1 and O_6 see Figure 3.1) were examined to determine the reliability of IQ scores.

(v) The relationship of children's IQ scores and their receptive and expressive language age scores were examined to determine predictability of the IQ scores in relation to either children's receptive, or expressive language development.

INTERNAL VALIDITY OF THE DESIGN

In general, internal validity checks whether the treatment variable (e.g. the experimental treatments X_2, X_3, X_4 and X_5) produced changes as reflected in the dependent variables. In order to claim that the independent variables do produce such changes it was necessary to check that some of the following extraneous variables have not produced an effect that can be mistaken for the effect of the experimental treatments.

74

The pre-test multiple post-test design has considerable internal validity due to:

(i) between test variations or contemporary history in or out of the experimental setting that occur between observation points O_1 to O_6, were controlled since they affected all groups from the same urban community equally;

(ii) the **within session variations** for the separate intervention and testing of groups were controlled because: (a) children were treated and tested individually; (b) children were randomly assigned to treatments wherever possible; (c) the testers for all pre and post-tests were randomly assigned to the subjects; (d) testers, whether for the criterion probes or for the standardised tests, were not informed as to which children were in particular treatment groups. Testers were not part of the distinct treatment programmes; (e) videotaping and independent observations of testing of individual teaching, and indeed in some instances normal classroom sessions, were an essential part of this programme. Therefore, it was possible to ascertain which children, if any, were receiving additional special attention in intact classrooms or clinic situations. Where this occurred then subjects have been excluded from the analysis; (f) The random assignment to groups, and the exclusion of subjects who had received unwanted attention, mean that situational factors have been controlled.

(iii) Biological and psychological **maturation** processes within the subjects have clearly changed during the progress of this three year experiment. Indeed, because of the time span of this research, and the number of testing situations for each experimental group it was possible to control and evaluate the effect of maturation upon the dependent variables.

(iv) The several tests given to all subjects over the period of the research may be regarded as affecting all groups equally. The fact that there were several tests provides more control over possible sources of internal invalidity than for a design in which the effect of **pre-testing** alone cannot be so controlled.

(v) Experimental mortality occurred in this research. However, 24 per cent of subjects given the original pre-tests, at O_1 (see above Figure 3.1 and p. 8) have been excluded from the final analysis. Thus, any differential loss which occurs if a particular subject drops out of a group after the experiment was underway was controlled, and this form of sampling bias was avoided.

(vi) Statistical **regression** was controlled as far as mean differences were concerned because all subjects were intellectually handicapped children and were randomly assigned to treatment groups. Therefore, although statistical regression occurred, it can safely be assumed that it occured equally with all groups.

(vii) Interaction of selection and history posed a problem in this study. The treatment X_1 was common for all groups and at this particular stage, no differential selection had taken place. However, some families resisted being placed in the Language Programme only Group D (see above p. 66) while others accepted their placement in this group. It must be noted, therefore, that Group D represented a non-volunteer group, certainly during Stage II, (see Figure 4.2 or from O_2 to O_5, Figure 3.1). This situation clearly may have affected parents' motivation. This must be accounted for in any explanation of differences between Group D and other treatment groups (see below Ch. 5 p. 100).

EXTERNAL VALIDITY OF THE DESIGN

External validity is concerned with the generalisability or representativeness of the experimental findings. The question is, do the results allow valid generalisations to other families and situations for which the subjects, settings and experimental variables of this study, were presumably representative? Can extraneous variables interact with the experimental treatment and make the subjects unrepresentative of the population of intellectually handicapped children? Can the claim be made, that the effect which treatments X_2, X_3, X_4 or X_5 (see above Figure 4.4 or Figure 3.1) had on the subjects, would be the same for other members of the population of intellectually handicapped children and their families who did not participate in this experiment?

PROBLEMS OF EXTERNAL VALIDITY

(i) **Interaction of pre-testing.** This particular design does not control for this possibility since all subjects receive the pre-tests at observation point O_1 (see above Figure 4.4 and Figure 3.1 p. 54). If the pre-testing sensitised or altered the subjects so that they responded differently than if no pre-testing had taken place, then the external validity would have been compromised. However, it is standard policy in Australian State and Territory Education Departments and Health Commission Assessment Clinics (T.A.C. 1980) for intellectually handicapped children to be regularly tested on standardised tests. Therefore, it can be assumed that the effect of pre-testing at observation point O_1 was representative. However, it should be noted that the *repeated* standardised tests and weekly criterion language checks (see (v) p. 73 above) may indeed compromise external validity.

(ii) **Reactive effects of the experimental treatments**
The experimental treatments may produce effects that limit the degree of generalization of the research findings. In this instance because the families knew they were in an experiment, then they may have reacted differently. For example, they may have made unusual efforts or co-operated to an unusual degree. Much emphasis was placed on the experimental nature of the treatment programmes, particularly the Target Teaching Group X_2 (see above Figure 3.1 and p. 58). This Target Teaching intervention had not been experienced before. All families knew that they were involved in a research programme and it was possible they acted atypically. For example, all parents completed Language Development Questionnaires (see above Ch. 3 & p. 56 and Appendix IV) during Stage I of the programme X_1 (Table 4.4). All children were given criterion language tests and the families in the treatment groups A, B and C were given additional backup and instructional materials. These changes could have affected the subjects' responses and thus, their relationship to other variables. This is the **Hawthorne effect** (Cooke, 1962) and explanations for this effect point to the factors; (a) novelty, and awareness that one is a participant in an experiment, (b) to a varified or modified environment involving special procedures and (c) new patterns of social interaction. As such, these factors created an awareness on the part of subjects which could become confounded with the independent variables under study (in this case the different treatment programmes or the different etiology groups), with a subsequent facilitating effect on the dependent variables, thus leading to ambiguous results. However, it was felt that the longitudinal nature of this programme and the different and distinct treatments X_1, X_2, X_3, X_4, X_5 or X_6 (see above Table 4.4) would be unlikely to bring about a consistent and sustained increase in effort by parents which *alone* would affect the measure of the dependent variables.

(iii) **Interaction of selection and treatments.** The characteristics of the families who participated in this experiment determine how extensively the research findings can be generalised. The children may be regarded as representative of any heterogeneous group of intellectually handicapped children even though they were not a random sample from a population of intellectually handicapped children, but, were rather a specific geographical sample. However, the socioeconomic status of their parents, as indicated by occupational structure (see Appendix VIII) had a greater proportion of persons in the professional and administrative classes than would be expected from a random selection of families with intellectually handicapped children. Therefore, this could compromise any generalisations made.

(iv) **Multiple-treatment inferences.** This longitudinal design exposed the subjects to, three or four different treatment procedures over the three years. This is shown below in Table 4.5.

Standardised testing and criterion language checks did take place at intervals between the different treatments. However, it may be difficult to effectively measure the effects of, for example, X_2 for Groups B and C when the influence of X_3 or X_4 was still effective. Hence, any generalisations regarding the effects of X_2 may be generalised only to Group A who experienced the same sequence of treatments X_2, X_2, X_2.

Hypotheses

In this research one particular experimental group and three other treatment groups were used. The intervention X_1 (see Tables 4.4 and 4.5 and Figure 3.1, p. 54) during Stage I was common and therefore the effects of independent variables, such as etiology, can be tested. Therefore, since the treatment X_1 was common, it was possible to directly study the effect of etiology on the dependent variables at observation points O_1 and O_2. The particular treatment interventions for Groups A, B and C during Stage II (see Figure 3.1) were absent from Group D. Therefore, any significant differences could be ascribed with confidence to the treatment X_2 Target Teaching, X_3 Social Work/Supportive Counselling or X_4 Speech Therapy, and to no other cause.

TABLE 4.5

Multiple Treatments for Experimental Groups

	Year 1	Year 2	Year 3
Group A	X_1	X_2, X_2, X_2	X_6
Group B	X_1	X_3, X_3, X_2	X_6
Group C	X_1	X_4, X_4, X_2	X_6
Group D	X_1	X_5, X_5, X_5	X_6

In the theory of hypothesis testing it is held that one of two "states of nature" may exist: either H_O (The Null Hypothesis) is true or H_1 (The Alternative Hypothesis) is true. H_1 constitutes the assertion that is accepted if H_O is rejected. Alternative hypotheses may be directional or non directional. As the literature on intervention studies is not sufficiently definitive to generate a high degree of confidence, bi-directional forms of alternative hypotheses were used.

Dependent variables for testing were the RRLA or RELA scores at observation points O_1, O_2, O_3, O_4, O_5 and O_6. In the testing of hypotheses to compare the effectiveness of the **sequence** of different treatments during the period O_2 to O_6 (see Fig. 3.1, p. 54), the multivariate F is based on a MANCOVA of the post-test scores at observation points O_3, O_4, O_5 and O_6. This overall analysis might be regarded as a rather conservative estimate of the treatment effects. This is because there were common treatments during Phase 3 from observation points O_4 to O_5 and throughout Stage III from observation points O_5 to O_6 (see Fig. 3.1 p. 54 and Table 4.4 p. 73). However, the purpose of this research was to examine the effectiveness of general service provision over time as well as the effectiveness of different treatments. Step down procedures were used to indicate the effectiveness of different treatments. Separate hypotheses for examining the effectiveness of sequences of treatments, using RRLA or RELA scores at observation points O_3, O_4, O_5 and O_6 and **particular** treatments, using RRLA or RELA scores at observation points O_3 and O_4, are presented. Other hypotheses examining the effects of sex and etiology on children's language development are based on a MANOVA of the RRLA or RELA scores at observation points O_1 to O_6 inclusive. As this research was exploratory the value of α was set at 0.05.

The Hypotheses: Eight sets of Hypotheses are presented.

HYPOTHESES FOR RECEPTIVE LANGUAGE TESTS

1. **Treatment Group Comparisons: Receptive Language Age Scores.**

   Hypothesis Ia That children in the Target Teaching Group perform differently on the Reynell Receptive Language Age Test at observation points O_3, O_4, O_5 and O_6 from children in the Social Work/Supportive Counselling Group B.

   Hypothesis Ib That children in the Target Teaching Group A perform differently on the Reynell Receptive Language Age Test at observation points O_3 and O_4 from children in the Social Work/Supportive Counselling Group B.

   Hypothesis Ic That children in the Target Teaching Group A perform differently on the Reynell Receptive Language Age Test at observation points O_3, O_4, O_5 and O_6 from children in the Speech Therapy Group C.

   Hypothesis Id That children in the Target Teaching Group A perform differently on the Reynell Receptive Language Age Test at observation points O_3 and O_4 from children in the Speech Therapy Group C.

   Hypothesis Ie That children in the Target Teaching Group A perform differently on the Reynell Receptive Language Age Test at observation points O_3, O_4, O_5 and O_6 from children in the Language Programme only Group D.

   Hypothesis If That children in the Target Teaching Group A perform differently on the Reynell Language Age Test, at observation points O_3 and O_4 from children in the Language Programme only Group D.

2. **Boys and Girls Comparisons: Receptive Language Age Scores.**

   Hypothesis IIa That all intellectually handicapped boys perform differently on the Reynell Receptive Language Age Test at observation points O_1, O_2, O_3, O_4, O_5 and O_6 from all intellectually handicapped girls.

3. **Etiology Group Comparisons: Receptive Language Age Scores.**

   Hypothesis IIIa That all Down's syndrome children perform differently on the Reynell Receptive Language Age Test at observation points O_1, O_2, O_3, O_4, O_5 and O_6 from all other intellectually handicapped children.

   Hypothesis IIIb That all Down's syndrome Children perform differently on the Reynell Receptive Language Age Test at observation points O_1, O_2, O_3, O_4, O_5 and O_6 from all children classified as Brain Damaged.

   Hypothesis IIIc That all Down's syndrome children perform differently on the Reynell Receptive Language Age Test at observation points O_1, O_2, O_3, O_4, O_5 and O_6 from children whose intellectual handicap is due to no known organic origin.

4. **Language Levels Comparison: Receptive Language Age Scores.**

   Hypothesis IVa That children at Language Level I in Target Teaching Group A perform differently on the Reynell Receptive Language Age Test at observation points O_3, O_4, O_5 and O_6 from children at Language Levels 2 and 3 in Target Teaching Group A.

   Hypothesis IVb That children at Language Level I in Social Work/Supportive Counselling Group B perform differently on the Reynell Receptive Language Age Test at observation points O_3, O_4, O_5 and O_6 from children at Language Levels 2 and 3 in Social Work/Supportive Counselling Group B.

   Hypothesis IVc That children at Language Level I in the Speech Therapy Group C perform differently on the Reynell Receptive Language Age Test at observation points O_3, O_4, O_5 and O_6 from children at Language Levels 2 and 3 in the Speech Therapy Group C.

   Hypothesis IV d That children at Language Level I in the Langage Programme only Group D perform differently on the Reynell Receptive Language Age Test at observation points O_3, O_4, O_5 and O_6 from children at Language Levels 2 and 3 in the Language Programme only Group D.

HYPOTHESES FOR EXPRESSIVE LANGUAGE TESTS

5. **Treatment Group Comparisons: Expressive Language Age Scores.**
   Hypothesis Va That children in Target Teaching Group A perform differently on the Reynell Expressive Language Age Test at observation points 0_3, 0_4, 0_5 and 0_6 from children in the Social Work/Supportive Counselling Group B.

   Hypothesis Vb That children in Target Teaching Group A perform differently on the Reynell Expressive Language Age Test at observation points 0_3 and 0_4 from children in the Social Work/Supportive Counselling Group B.

   Hypothesis Vc That children in Target Teaching Group A perform differently on the Reynell Expressive Language Age Test at observation points 0_3, 0_4, 0_5 and 0_6 from children in the Speech Therapy Group C.

   Hypothesis Vd That children in Target Teaching Group A perform differently on the Reynell Expressive Language Age Test at observation points 0_3 and 0_4 from children in the Speech Therapy Group C.

   Hypothesis Ve That children in the Target Teaching Group A perform differently on the Reynell Expressive Language Age Test at observation points 0_3, 0_4, 0_5 and 0_6 from children in the Language Programme only Group D.

   Hypothesis Vf That children in the Target Teaching Group A perform differently on the Reynell Expressive Language Age Test at observation points 0_3 and 0_4 from children in the Language Programme only Group D.

6. **Boys and Girls Comparison: Expressive Language Age Scores.**
   Hypothesis VI That all intellectually handicapped boys perform differently on the Reynell Expressive Language Age Test at observation points 0_1, 0_2, 0_3, 0_4, 0_5 and 0_6 from all intellectually handicapped girls.

7. **Etiology Group Comparisons: Expressive Language Age Scores.**
   Hypothesis VIIa That all Down's Syndrome children perform differently on the Reynell Expressive Language Age Test at observation points 0_1, 0_2, 0_3, 0_4, 0_5 and 0_6 from all other intellectually handicapped children.

   Hypothesis VIIb That all Down's Syndrome children perform differently on the Reynell Expressive Language Age Test at observation points 0_1, 0_2, 0_3, 0_4, 0_5 and 0_6 from all children classified as Brain Damaged.

   Hypothesis VIIc That all Down's Syndrome children perform differently on the Reynell Expressive Language Age Test at observation points 0_1, 0_2, 0_3, 0_4, 0_5 and 0_6 from children whose intellectual handicap is due to no known organic origin.

8. **Language Levels Comparisons: Expressive Language Age Scores.**
   Hypothesis VIIIa That children at Language Level I, in Target Teaching Group A perform differently on the Reynell Expressive Language Age Test at observation points 0_3, 0_4, 0_5 and 0_6 from children at Language Levels 2 and 3 in Target Teaching Group A.

   Hypothesis VIIIb That children at Language Level I in the Social Work/Supportive Counselling Group B perform differently on the Reynell Expressive Language Age Test at observation points 0_3, 0_4, 0_5 and 0_6 from children at Language Levels 2 and 3 in the Social Work/Supportive Counselling Group B.

   Hypothesis VIIIc That children at Language Level I in the Speech Therapy Group C perform differently on the Reynell Expressive Language Age Test at observation points 0_3, 0_4, 0_5 and 0_6 from children at Language Levels 2 and 3 in the Speech Therapy Group C.

   Hypothesis VIIId That children at Language Level I in the Language Programme only Group D perform differently on the Reynell Expressive Language Age Test at observation points 0_3, 0_4, 0_5 and 0_6 from children at Language Levels 2 and 3 in the Language Programme only Group D.

PART TWO

THE RESULTS

Chapter Five

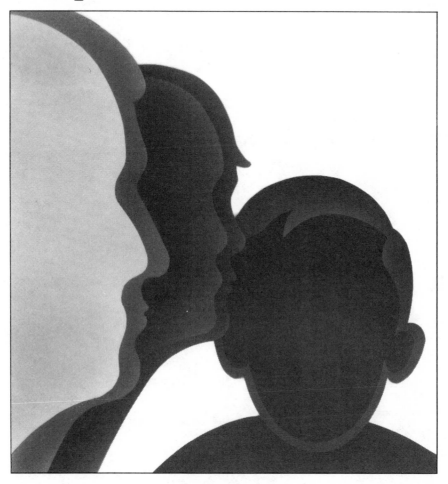

Language Acquisition and
IQ Score/Results

RECEPTIVE LANGUAGE RESULTS

Preliminary Considerations

Understanding simple and then more complex commands and questions, can be achieved by the intellectually handicapped when a teaching programme comprises a series of small steps. These small steps begin, with teaching eye contact and attention getting procedures. This is followed by teaching non-verbal responses which provide feedback so that the listener can indicate that he or she is, or is not understanding. Then follows the teaching of gestural and verbal responses to commands and questions. In this teaching programme, facial, body and verbal cues and clues are given in the early stages to help the child always make the correct response. The receptive language measures used in this programme, are an indication, of children's ability to respond to these teaching procedures and in so doing comprehend what is said.

One of the main problems with the Reynell Verbal Comprehension Scale, used here with the intellectually handicapped, was that there was always the chance that the children were responding to the whole complex of communications of which the actual spoken instructions was only one element. The teaching and assessment of children with receptive language disorders is at an early stage and it is easy to credit children with a greater degree of language comprehension than is readily available to them.

A further problem that must be considered before interpreting these results, is, that there is little agreement as to whether the receptive language delay of these children is essentially one of quantity, or of quality. This dispute is of relevance in a discussion on the longitudinal effects of different treatment programmes. For example, Carrow-Woolfolk (1975) argues that severely language delayed children are different from rather than slower than normal children. However, Morehead and Ingram (1973) argue that the difference between children who are significantly delayed in verbal comprehension and normal children is essentially quantitative. Eisenson (1980) states that this issue is more determined by the bias of the investigator than by the achievements of the child. For example, both the quantity and quality of an intellectually handicapped child's language can be directly influenced by different teaching strategies and goals. In this setting the teacher or therapist can exercise a powerful effect on a child's language development by systematically varying different aspects of the teaching situation. For example, if an aim of teaching is to increase a child's understanding of increasing numbers of named objects then correct responses to different named objects would be taught. If the aim is to teach an understanding of verbs then the teaching situation could use pictures depicting different activities. If the aim is to develop an understanding of subject, verb and object, then pictures depicting subject, verb, object relationships would be used.

What seems clear is that when the quantity of language a child understands reaches a certain amount, for example a number of objects correctly identified, then this effect is qualitative. Witness the "take-off" at 18 months referred to by Menyuk (1976), Bloom and Lahey (1978) Hopper and Naremore (1978). Parents of the intellectually handicapped look for and often long for this "take-off". Therefore which teaching or treatment programme will enable these children to develop strategies of comprehension, for how long these teaching programmes should be applied, which group of intellectually handicapped children or which age level will intervention be most effective for, are recurring questions for parents.

Receptive Language Results as measured by the Reynell Developmental Language Scale, Verbal Comprehension Test (RRLA).

Comparison of Treatment Groups.

1. Group A vs. Group B.

Children in the experimental Target Teaching Group A (see Tables 5.1 and 5.2 and Fig. 5.1) showed a greater improvement in Reynell Receptive Language Age (RRLA) scores over the periods of intervention 0_2 to 0_3 and or the period 0_2 to 0_6 (see Table 5.2).

TABLE 5.1

Reynell Receptive Language Age (R R L A) Estimated* amd Adjusted[ø] Mean Scores for Different Treatment Groups

Group	N	Pre-test Mean O_1	Pre-test Mean O_2	Post-test Mean O_3	Adjusted Post-test Mean O_3	Post-test Mean O_4	Adjusted Post-test Mean O_4	Post-test Mean O_5	Adjusted Post-test Mean O_5	Post-test Mean O_6	Adjusted Post-test Mean O_6
A	25	27.8	30.20	36.30	37.9	37.1	38.6	38.5	39.6	40.9	42.3
B	24	26.3	26.70	28.9	33.9	29.6	34.9	32.7	37.5	33.5	38.2
C	25	23.9	24.50	25.9	33.3	27.4	35.1	27.7	34.6	29.4	36.1
D	28	25.9	28.1	29.2	32.9	30.0	33.7	30.1	33.2	29.6	32.9

* Estimated mean R R L A scores based on a MANOVA analysis of observed scores at observation points O_1, O_2, O_3, O_4, O_5 and O_6.

ø Adjusted mean R R L A scores O_3 to O_6 inclusive based on a MANCOVA analysis using R R L A scores at observation points O_1 and O_2 as covariates.

FIG. 5.1

Graphical Representation of Mean Reynell Receptive Language Age Scores & Adjusted Post-Test Scores in Treatment Groups

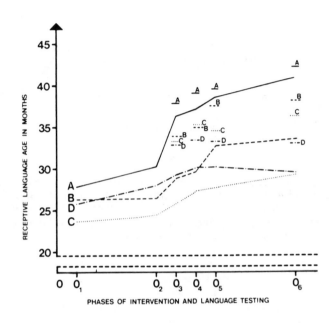

ADJUSTED SCORES

————— A   Target Teaching Group A
- - - - - B   Social Work/Supportive Counselling Group B
················· C   Speech Therapy Group C
—·—·—·— D   Language Programme Only Group D

87

TABLE 5.2

Percentage R R L A Gains for Each Treatment Group During Successive
Phases of Intervention ø

Group	% gain 0_2 to 0_3	% gain 0_3 to 0_4	% gain 0_4 to 0_5	% gain 0_5 to 0_6	Overall % gain 0_2 to 0_6
A	20.0	2.0	4.0	6.0	35.0
B	8.0	3.0	10.0	2.0	25.0
C	6.0	6.0	1.0	6.0	20.0
D	4.0	3.0	-	-	5.0

ø Percentage gains based on estimated R R L A mean scores. Estimated
mean scores calculated by using a MANOVA of the R R L A observed
scores 0_1 to 0_6 inclusive.

(Cooper Moodley and Reynell (1979) report a "40 per cent progress"
in R R L A scores over a period of 5 years for the 10 intellectually
handicapped children (non verbal I Q of <65) in their study. Group
A children in this study achieved a 20 per cent gain in R R L A
scores during the first three months of Target Teaching.)

However, multivariate analysis of covariance (MANCOVA) indicated that the difference
between the mean RRLA scores for children in Group A and Group B at observation points 0_3,
0_4, 0_5 and 0_6 was not statistically significant F=1.115, df=4 and 40, p<0.36. Likewise the
difference between the mean RRLA scores for children in Group A and Group B at observation
points 0_3 and 0_4 was not statistically significant (see Table 5.3).

TABLE 5.3

Probability Levels for Univariate and Step Down F Values when R R L A
Mean Scores for Groups A & B were Compared   at Observation Points
0_3 and 0_4.

Variable	Error Mean Square	Hypothesis Mean Square	Univariate F	P Less Than	Step Down F	P Less Than
RRLA 0_3	9.983	5.61	0.56	0.4576	0.56	0.4576
RRLA 0_4	19.002	22.87	1.20	0.2787	0.64	0.4299

2. Group A vs. Group C.
    Children in the experimental Target Teaching Group A (see Tables 5.1 and 5.2 and Fig.
5.1) showed a greater improvement in RRLA scores over the periods of intervention 0_2 to 0_3 and

0_2 to 0_6 than children in the Speech Therapy Group C (see Table 5.2). However, a MANCOVA indicated that the difference between the mean RRLA scores for children in Group A and Group C at observation points 0_3, 0_4, 0_5 and 0_6 was not statistically significant ($F=1.343$ df=4 and 40, $p<0.271$). Likewise the difference between the mean RRLA scores for children in Group A and Group C at observation points 0_3 and 0_4 was not statistically significant (see Table 5.4).

TABLE 5.4

Probability Levels for Univariate and Step Down F Values when R R L A Mean Scores for Groups A & C were Compared ø at Observation Points 0_3 and 0_4.

Variable	Error Mean Square	Hypothesis Mean Square	Univariate F	P Less Than	Step Down F	P Less Than
RRLA 0_3	9.983	32.89	3.29	0.0765	3.29	0.0765
RRLA 0_4	19.002	3.07	0.16	0.6898	2.07	0.1581

ø Based on MANCOVA with pre-tests R R L A at observation points 0_1 and 0_2 as covariates. R R L A: Reynell Receptive Language Age.

3. Group A vs. Group D.

Children in the experimental Target Teaching Group A (see Tables 5.1 and 5.2 and Fig. 5.1) showed a considerably greater improvement in RRLA scores over the periods of intervention 0_2 to 0_3 and 0_2 to 0_6 then children in the Language Programme only Group D (see Table 5.2). MANCOVA of the RRLA scores at observation points 0_3, 0_4, 0_5 and 0_6 indicated that there was a statistically significant difference between the mean RRLA scores for children in Group A and children in Group D. ($F=6.864$ df=4 and 40.0, $p<0.0003$).

TABLE 5.5

Probability Levels for Univariate and Step Down F Values when R R L A Mean Scores for Groups A and D were Compared ø at Observation Points 0_3, 0_4, 0_5 and 0_6.

Variable	Error Mean Square	Hypothesis Mean Square	Univariate F	P Less Than	Step Down F	P Less Than
RRLA 0_3	9.983	239.98	23.74	0.0001	23.74	0.0001
RRLA 0_4	19.002	257.33	13.54	0.0007	0.0011	0.97
RRLA 0_5	114.69	456.61	3.98	0.0524	0.33	0.57
RRLA 0_6	64.11	946.02	14.76	0.0004	3.11	0.09

ø Based on MANCOVA with pre-tests R R L A at observation points 0_1 and 0_2 as covariates. R R L A: Reynell Receptive Language Age.

89

Examination of the step-down F tests (see Table 5.5) indicated that it was at the end of phase I (see Fig. 3.1 p. 54) at observation point O_3 after three months of Target Teaching that there was a statistically significant difference between the adjusted RRLA scores of children in the experimental Target Teaching Group A and the adjusted RRLA scores of children in the Language Programme only Group D. (Step down $F=23.74$ $p<0.0001$).

4. Comparison of Boys and Girls: Receptive Language Age Scores.

Boys showed a slightly greater improvement in mean scores over the time period O_1 to O_6 (see Table 5.6). Over the period of the interventions O_2 to O_6 (see Table 5.4) the per centage gains in RRLA scores for boys and girls were both 18 per cent. A Multivariate analysis of variance (MANOVA) of the RRLA scores, at observation points O_1, O_2, O_3, O_4, O_5 and O_6 indicated that there was no statistical difference between the mean RRLA scores for boys and girls ($F=0.534$ df=6 and 40.0 $p<0.779$). Similarly, a MANOVA of the RRLA scores at observation points O_3, O_4, O_5 and O_6 following the specific interventions indicated again that there was no statistically significant difference between the mean RRLA scores for boys and girls ($F=0.701$ df=4 and 42.0 $p<0.596$).

Comparison of Etiology Groups: Receptive Language Age Scores.

5. Downs' Syndrome Children vs. All Other Intellectually Handicapped Children.

Downs' syndrome children showed a greater improvement in RRLA scores than all the other intellectually handicapped children in the programme (see Table 5.7). However, a MANOVA of the RRLA scores at observation points O_1, O_2, O_3, O_4, O_5 and O_6 indicated that there was no statistically significant difference between the mean RRLA scores for Downs' syndrome children and all other intellectually handicapped children ($F=1.727$ df=4 and 42.0 $p<0.162$).

6. Downs' Syndrome vs. Brain Damaged Children.

Downs' syndrome children showed a slightly greater improvement in RRLA scores over the total period of the programme O_1 to O_6 (see Table 5.7). A 30 per cent gain in mean RRLA scores was achieved by the Downs' syndrome children whereas the children classified as Brain Damaged achieved a 27 per cent gain overall. However, there were periods in the programme for example from O_3 to O_4 and O_4 to O_5 when the Brain Damaged children showed greater RRLA gain scores (see again Table 5.7). However, a MANOVA of the RRLA scores throughout the period of the programme O_1 to O_6 indicated that there was no positively significant difference between the mean RRLA scores for Down's syndrome children and children classified as Brain Damaged ($F=1.062$ df=6 and 40.0 $p< 0.401$). Similarly a MANOVA of the RRLA scores at observation points O_3, O_4, O_5 and O_6 following the specific interventions again indicated that there was no statistically significant difference between the mean RRLA scores for Down's syndrome children and all children classified as Brain Damaged ($F=0.596$, df=4 and 42.0 $p< 0.668$).

7. Down's Syndrome vs. Mentally Handicapped. ♂

Down's syndrome children showed a considerably greater improvement in RRLA scores than children whose intellectual handicap was due to no known origin (see Table 5.7). For example, Down's syndrome children achieved a 30 per cent gain in mean RRLA scores from O_1 to O_6 whereas the children whose intellectual handicap was due to no known organic origin only achieved a gain of 18 per cent. However, when the RRLA gains were examined for the period O_2 to O_6 following the specific interventions, then the advantage achieved by the Down's syndrome children was considerably reduced. For example, Down's syndrome children achieved a 23 per cent gain in mean RRLA scores fro O_2 to O_6, whereas, the children whose intellectual handicap was due to no known organic origin achieved a 19 per cent gain.

♂ Mentally Handicapped: Children whose intellectual handicap is due to no known organic origin.

TABLE 5.6

Mean Reynell Receptive Language Age Scores in Months ø for Boys and Girls
During the Period O_1 to O_6 and Per Centage Gains in R R L A Scores in Each Time Period

	N	C.A. at O_1 mths.	RRLA at O_1	RRLA at O_2	% Gain O_1 to O_2	RRLA at O_3	% Gain O_2 to O_3	RRLA at O_4	% Gain O_3 to O_4	RRLA at O_5	% Gain O_4 to O_5	RRLA at O_6	% Gain O_5 to O_6	% Gain O_1 to O_6	% Gain O_2 to O_6
All Boys	58	72	30.7	32.3	8.0	34.9	8.0	35.3	1.0	36.6	4.0	38.0	4.0	24.0	18.0
All Girls	44	62	30.3	31.0	2.0	33.8	9.0	34.8	3.0	36.4	5.0	36.5	-	20.0	18.0

ø Estimated mean R R L A scores obtained by using a MANOVA analysis of the observed R R L A mean scores O_1 to O_6 inclusive.

TABLE 5.7

Reynell Receptive Language Age Mean Scores ∅ in Months for Different Etiology Groups

During the Period O_1 to O_6 and Per Centage Gains in R R L A Scores in Each Time Period

Etiology Group	N	Mean CA at O_1 Mths.	RRLA at O_1	RRLA at O_2	% gain O_1 to O_2	RRLA at O_3	% gain O_2 to O_3	RRLA at O_4	% gain O_3 to O_4	RRLA at O_5	% gain O_4 to O_5	RRLA at O_6	% gain O_5 to O_6	% gain O_1 to O_6	% gain O_2 to O_6
Down's Syndrome	57	63	28.0	29.6	6.0	32.7	10.0	33.1	1.0	34.7	5.0	36.4	5.0	30.0	23.0
All other M.H. children	45	72	30.9	32.0	4.0	34.7	8.0	35.4	2.0	36.8	4.0	37.4	2.0	21.0	17.0
Brain Damaged	16	75	29.2	30.1	3.0	31.3	4.0	32.5	4.0	36.0	11.0	36.7	2.0	27.0	22.0
Mentally Handi-capped *	10	98	38.1	37.6	-1.0	40.7	8.0	41.2	1.0	42.7	4.0	44.8	5.0	18.0	19.0

∅ Estimated mean R R L A scores obtained by using a MANOVA analysis of the observed R R L A scores for the period O_1 to O_6.

* Mentally handicapped: children whose mental handicap is due to no known organic origin.

MANOVA of the RRLA scores throughout the period of the programme O_1 to O_6 indicated that there was a statistically significant difference between the mean RRLA scores for Down's syndrome children and children whose intellectual handicap was due to no known origin ($F=3.336$ df=6 and 40.0 p< 0.009). Examination of the step-down F tests derived from the MANOVA of the RRLA scores O_1 to O_6 (see Table 5.8) showed that it was at O_1 that the step-down F value was statistically significant (Step-down $F=20.219$ P< 0.0001). However, a MANOVA of the RRLA scores at observation points O_3, O_4, O_5 and O_6 following the specific interventions indicated that there was no statistically significant difference between the mean RRLA scores for Down's syndrome children and children whose intellectual handicap was due to no known organic origin ($F=1.464$, df=4 and 42, p< 0.23). It is felt that this is most pertinent and is referred to in the discussion on receptive language results below (p. 100).

TABLE 5.8

Probability Levels for Univariate and Step Down F Values when Mean R R L A Scores at Observation Points O_1, O_2, O_3, O_4, O_5 and O_6 were Compared ø1 for Down's Syndrome Children and Mentally Handicapped Children ø2.

Variable	Error Mean Square	Hypothesis Mean Square	Univariate F	P Less Than	Step Down F	P Less Than
RRLA O_1	38.765	783.80	20.22	0.0001	2C.22	0.0001
RRLA O_2	76.211	507.82	6.66	0.0132	1.19	0.28
RRLA O_3	86.424	494.30	5.72	0.0211	0.09	0.77
RRLA O_4	107.136	508.65	4.75	0.0347	0.01	0.90
RRLA O_5	195.762	503.55	2.57	0.1158	0.09	0.77
RRLA O_6	131.817	557.82	4.23	0.0455	0.14	0.71

Comparison of Language Levels within Treatment Groups: Receptive

ø1 Based on MANOVA of R R L A scores at observation points O_1 to O_6.
ø2 Mentally Handicapped Children: Children whose intellectual handicap is due to no known organic origin.

Comparison of Etiology Groups: Receptive Language Age Scores

8. Experimental Target Teaching Group A Level I vs Levels 2 and 3.
The advantage in mean RRLA gain scores favoured children at Language Level I (see Tables 5.9, 5.10 and 5.11). The difference between the mean estimated RRLA scores of children at different language levels was statistically significant no matter whether a MANOVA of RRLA scores at observation points O_1, O_2, O_3, O_4, O_5 and O_6 was calculated ($F=22.982$ df =6 and 40.0 p< 0.0001) or a MANOVA of RRLA scores at observation points O_3, O_4, O_5 and O_6 following the specific intervention was calculated ($F=13.842$, df=4 and 42.0, p< 0.0001). However, the distribution of children into different language levels pre-supposed an initial distinct difference in language age scores. This was confirmed. The aim was to examine whether the success of an intervention was dependent on a child's level of language acquisition at the commencement of the intervention.

TABLE 5.9

Reynell Receptive Language Age Mean Scores ∅ O_1 to O_6 for Language Levels within Treatment Groups

GROUP	Language Level	N	Mean CA at O_1 in Months	S.D. in Months	O_1 RRLA	O_2 RRLA	O_3 RRLA	O_4 RRLA	O_5 RRLA	O_6 RRLA
A	1	12	42.3	17.8	13.3	16.5	23.3	24.4	25.7	30.5
	2 & 3	13	80.8	28.5	42.3	43.9	49.4	49.8	51.3	51.4
B	1	12	56.7	30.0	12.8	13.7	16.1	17.1	18.7	18.3
	2 & 3	12	85.0	34.8	39.8	39.7	41.6	42.2	46.6	48.6
C	1	13	44.6	15.4	11.3	13.0	14.2	16.4	15.7	18.3
	2 & 3	12	97.2	31.6	36.6	35.9	37.6	38.4	39.7	40.4
D	1	13	51.3	11.3	11.8	15.0	15.7	17.4	17.9	19.3
	2 & 3	15	84.3	28.7	39.8	41.3	42.7	42.5	42.4	40.0

∅ Estimated mean R R L A scores obtained by using a MANOVA analysis of the observed R R L A scores for the period O_1 to O_6.

Language Level 1 refers to children whose combined Reynell Developmental Language Age (R D L A) at O_1 was 18 months or less.

Language Levels 2 & 3 refer to children whose combined Reynell Developmental Language Age (R D L A) was greater than 18 months at O_1.

TABLE 5.10

Per Centage R R L A Gains for Language Levels Within Treatment Groups Following Each Period of Intervention

GROUP	Language Level	N	% Gain O_1 to O_2	% Gain O_2 to O_3	% Gain O_3 to O_4	% Gain O_4 to O_5	% Gain O_5 to O_6	% Gain O_1 to O_6	% Gain O_2 to O_6
A	1	12	24.1	41.2	4.7	5.3	18.7	129.3	84.8
	2 & 3	13	3.8	12.5	1.0	3.0	-	21.5	17.1
B	1	12	7.0	17.5	6.2	9.4	-2.0	43.0	33.6
	2 & 3	12	-	5.0	1.4	10.4	4.3	22.1	22.4
C	1	13	15.0	9.2	15.5	-4.3	16.6	61.9	40.8
	2 & 3	12	-1.9	4.7	2.1	3.4	1.8	10.4	12.5
D	1	15	27.1	10.5	10.8	2.9	7.8	63.6	28.7
	2 & 3	15	10.4	10.3	-0.5	-0.2	-5.7	0.5	-3.1

ø Per centage gains calculated from estimated mean R R L A scores.

Estimated mean R R L A scores obtained by using a MANOVA analysis of the observed R R L A scores for the period O_1 to O_6.

Language Level 1 refers to children with a combined Reynell Developmental Language Age of less than 18 months at O_1.

Language Levels 2 & 3 refer to children with a combined Reynell Developmental Language Age of 18 months and above at O_1.

TABLE 5.11

Reynell Receptive Language Age Adjusted Mean Scores ∅ O_3 to O_6

For Language Levels Within Treatment Groups Following Each Period of Intervention

GROUP	Language Level	N	Adj. R R L A at O_3	Adj. R R L A at O_4	Adj. R R L A at O_5	Adj. R R L A at O_6
A	1	12	38.8	40.6	39.6	44.6
	2 & 3	13	36.9	36.7	39.6	39.9
B	1	12	34.5	36.3	35.8	35.2
	2 & 3	12	33.3	33.6	39.3	41.1
C	1	13	33.4	33.6	39.3	41.1
	2 & 3	12	33.1	33.8	36.0	36.4
D	1	13	32.9	35.3	33.3	34.9
	2 & 3	15	32.9	32.1	33.1	30.9

∅ Adjusted mean R R L A scores O_3 to O_6 based on a MANCOVA analysis using observed R R L A scores at O_1 to O_2 as covariates. Language Level 1 refers to children with a combined Reynell Developmental Language Age of less than 18 months at O_1. Language Levels 2 and 3 refer to children with a combined Reynell Developmental Language Age of 18 months and above at O_1.

Therefore a MANCOVA of the RRLA scores at observation points O_3, O_4, O_5 and O_6 was computed with RRLA observed scores at observation points O_1 and O_2 as covariates. This MANCOVA analysis indicated that there was no statistically significant difference between the adjusted mean RRLA scores (see Table 5.11) for children at Language Level I (with a combined Reynell Developmental Language Age RDLA score at or below 18 months at observation point O_1) and the adjusted mean RRLA scores (see Table 5.11) for children at Language Levels 2 and 3 (with a combined RDLA score above 18 months at observation point O_1), ($F=0.382$ df=4 and 40.0 p< 0.821).

9. Social Work/Supportive Counselling Group B. Language Level 1 vs. Language Levels 2 and 3.

The advantage in mean RRLA gain scores, as indicated by per centage RRLA gains, overall favours children at language level 1 (see Tables 5.9 and 5.10). However, during time periods O_4 to O_5 (when the specific Target Teaching programme was applied to Group B) and from O_5 to O_6 the advantage in per centage RRLA gains slightly favoured children at language levels 2 and 3. A MANOVA of the RRLA scores throughout the period of the program O_1 to O_6 indicated that, there was a statistically significant difference between the mean scores for children at Language Level 1 (with a combined Reynell Developmental Language Age (RDLA) score at or below 18 months at O_1) and children at Language Levels 2 and 3 (with a combined RDLA score about 18 months at O_1) $F=16.695$ df=6 and 40.0 p< 0.0001). Likewise a MANOVA of the RRLA scores at observation points O_3, O_4, O_5 and O_6 (see above Fig. 3.1 p. 54) indicated that there was also a statistically significant difference between the mean RRLA scores for children at Language Level 1 and the mean RRLA scores for children at Language Levels 2 and 3 ($F=12.112$ df=4 and 42, p<0.0001).

However, a MANCOVA of the RRLA scores at observation points O_3, O_4, O_5 and O_6 with RRLA scores at observation points O_1 and O_2 as covariates indicated that there was no statistically significant difference between the adjusted mean RRLA scores (see Table 5.11) for children at Language Level 1 and the adjusted mean RRLA score (see Table 5.9) for children at Language Levels 2 and 3 ($F=0.797$, df=4 and 40.0 p<0.535).

10. Speech Therapy Group C. Language Level 1 vs. Language Levels 2 & 3.

The advantage in mean RRLA gain scores clearly favoured children at Language Level 1 (see Tables 5.9 and 5.10). The difference between the mean estimated RRLA scores of children at different language levels was statistically significant no matter whether a MANOVA of RRLA scores at observation points O_1, O_2, O_3, O_4, O_5 and O_6 was calculated ($F=15.197$ df=6 and 40.0 p<0.0001).

However, a MANCOVA of the RRLA scores at observation points O_3, O_4, O_5 and O_6 with RRLA scores at O_1 and O_2 as covariates indicated that there was no statistically significant difference between the adjusted mean RRLA scores (see Table 5.11) for children at Language Level 1 (with a combined RDLA score at or below 18 months at O_1) and the adjusted mean RRLA scores (see Table 5.11) for children at Language Levels 2 and 3 (with a combined RDLA score above 18 months at O_1) ($F=0.427$, df=4 and 40.0 p<0.788).

11. Language Programme Only Group D. Language Level 1 vs. language Levels 2 & 3.

Once again the advantage in mean RRLA gain scores clearly favoured children at Language Level 1 (see Table 5.9, 5.10 and 5.11). The difference between the mean estimated RRLA scores of children at different language levels was again, as anticipated, statistically significant no matter whether a MANOVA of RRLA scores at observation points O_1, O_2, O_3, O_4, O_5 and O_6 was calculated ($F=21.239$, df=6 and 40.0 p<0.0001) or whether a MANOVA of RRLA scores at observation points O_3, O_4, O_5 and O_6 following the introduction of a written language program was calculated ($F=15.917$ df=4 and 42 p<0.0001).

However, a MANCOVA of the RRLA scores at observation points O_3, O_4, O_5 and O_6 with RRLA scores at observation points O_1 and O_2 as covariates indicated that there was no statistically significant difference between the adjusted mean RRLA scores (see Table 5.11) for children at Language Level 1 and the adjusted mean RRLA scores (see Table 5.11) for children at Language Levels 2 and 3 ($F=0.569$, df=4 and 40.0 p<0.686).

Discussion of Receptive Language Results.

Different Treatment Programmes

The results, of the effects, of the different interventions on the development of children's measured receptive language in the present study indicated the following:

(i) that the provision of a structured behaviourally-based language teaching programme, similar to that developed by Sailor, Guess and Baer (1973) and Kent (1972), along with regular teaching by parents, was significantly more effective than the mere provision to parents of just that written behaviourally-based language teaching programme. However, it was not significantly more effective than providing parents with the behaviourally-based written programme plus regular guidance from social workers or counsellors, or providing parents with the behaviourally-based written programme and back-up developmental speech therapy services. This finding contrasts with that of Heifetz (1977) who found that providing parents with a behaviourally-based instructional manual "packaged for parents of retarded children" was as effective as the professional involvement formats. However, it should be pointed out that Heifetz's programme was only trialled for 20 weeks;

(ii) that the greatest mean gains[ø] in measured receptive language ages occurred in the initial three months of the application of Target Teaching. This occurred during Phase 1 O_2 to O_3 for the experimental Target Teaching Group A (a mean gain of 6.10 months with a range −1 to +15 months) and during Phase III O_4 to O_5 for Group B (a mean gain of 3.10 months with a range −6 to +22 months). It is pertinent to note when the greatest initial gains occurred for it confirmed the findings of Bidder, Bryant and Gray (1975) that it is **early** in a structured intervention (the first 2 months in their case) that improvements in receptive language behaviours or behaviours related to verbal comprehension are noticed. They point out that the early rate of progress (as measured in the Griffiths Developmental Scale, Griffiths 1964) "was not likely to be maintained". Similarly, Sajwaj (1973) pointed out that for the behavioural technique to be used effectively then "regular external prompts were required". When these external prompts were removed **later** in training then the interventions became less and less effective as "the parents' level of attention slowly dropped back to what was normal for them prior to the behavioural intervention". Therefore, while the greatest improvement in children's comprehension can be expected to occur in the first few months of a behaviourally oriented intervention, it is to be expected that progress will not be maintained at the initial rate (see Fig. 5.1). This view is supported clearly by findings in this research;

(iii) that it was children in the experimental Target Teaching Group A who achieved most improvement in receptive language ages during the **final** phase of the intervention O_5 to O_6 (see Fig. 5.1 and Tables 5.1 and 5.2). This "maintained improvement" by children in Group A provided relevant information for parents. The Target Teaching programme was designed to teach parents strategies for developing and maintaining their children's receptive language skills. Maintaining receptive language gains over longer periods was different operationally than achieving gains in the initial phase of intervention. This was because:

(a) parent motivation and persistence in the short term (a period of 3 months) may be reinforced by evidence of their children's improved comprehension (see Fig. 5.1 and Table 5.2), but, in the long term, (9 months and more) this evidence may not be so obvious and therefore other factors such as family and group cohesion may be required to encourage parents to persevere with teaching;

(b) the length of time parents and professionals spent together helped determine group support and cohesion. Therefore, the longer the period of training, the greater was the likelihood of group cohesion and parents' perseverance;

(c) that willingness to persevere with learning a skill (e.g. teaching relevant understanding)

ø   These mean receptive language age gains ignored the fact that the children were 3 months older at the end of each phase of intervention.

...tion of critical periods for the intellectually handicapped to develop
...skills was examined. Is there a language age in which there are period...
...itivities to interventions, or particular response propensities which can be fu...
...e appeared to be a chronological sequence of language acquisition which suppor...
...1965) and Elkind's (1974) position. Furthermore, the sequence of comprehension...
...ounded by these children's developmental levels and as such would seem to support
...6) and Vygotsky's (1962) position regarding the egocentrism of both language and
...wever, the proposition that a child's **level** of receptive language will be likely to
...he effectiveness of interventions also depends on the evidence that: (a) there are
...rts and plateaus in the rate of acquisitions of comprehension skills and that the
...ss of an intervention may be determined by whether the intervention coincides with a
...urt" or "plateau" or that (b) the older intellectually handicapped child has more
...eviance, or less effective comprehension strategies due to indifferent learning and is
...o benefit from interventions than the younger child. This proposition assumes that the
...ld presents quite deficient comprehension strategies and that these have to be
...d, before improvement can accrue, or be noticed. It is a proposition that assumes a
...on of language experiences similar to those that have been demonstrated to exist in
...nal environments (Lyle 1959, Melyn and White 1973). Careful study of children in this
...me (see Chapters 1 and 3) indicated that there was no evidence of language deprivation
...homes that was comparable with that observed in institutions.
...he results of this study of the acquisition of receptive language skills by intellectually
...apped children at different language levels within treatment groups illustrated that:
...ere was no evidence of different rates of receptive language acquisition by children
...ommencing at different levels of measured receptive language skills within the same
...eatment group.
...here was no evidence of older children living at home having less effective comprehension
...trategies than younger children. It seems therefore, that if the home environment a lá
...Johnson (1979) is similar then there is every reason to believe that the older child is **as** open
...to learning new comprehension skills as the younger child. However, it was considered that
...there were no children in this study who were sufficiently old enough to support Lenneberg's
...position that "progress in language learning comes to a halt after maturity". A further
...longitudinal study is required to confirm this question of reduced sensitivity to language
...stimulation after a certain age.
...) there was no evidence, from children in these different treatment groups, of a particular time
...of onset of comprehension skills, or of their termination. Rather, there was some evidence of a
...plateauing effect (see Tables 5.9 and 5.10) which, if the study were continued, might prove to
...be the springboard for further language development as recognised by Beveridge, Spencer &
...Mittler (1978) and Swann and Mittler (1976).

EXPRESSIVE LANGUAGE RESULTS

Preliminary Considerations:

The assessment of expressive language in Carrow's terms (Carrow 1972) is concerned with
observing: the production of reflexive sound utterances which are indicated by a child's ability to
cry, to babble, and otherwise to produce voice and articulate sounds; secondly, it is concerned
with the role of automatic speech in which accurate sounds and words in appropriate sequence
are produced. Accordingly, children who function well at this level, are considered, to be able to
demonstrate good association between the auditory and vocal systems. This association may be
indicated by a child's ability to imitate well. A higher level skill, which may be regarded as akin to
Reynell's "Creative use of language", is meaningful formulation and speech production. This
skill shows that speech not only has meaning, but also that new meanings are coded by the child,
in order that he or she may express them.

meant that there was a greater chance of that skill becoming part of a child's domestic
routine and of that skill being encoded in memory;

(d) comprehension often depended on multiple cued behaviour (see Ch. 8 p. 195) and
required analysis not merely in terms of the sending and receiving of messages but also
analysis of comprehension as a piece of social behaviour. These social skills must be
planned in the sense that they have to be taught, reinforced and hopefully, maintained
and generalised. The procedural control that Zifferblatt observes as necessary for the
teaching of a skill (Zifferblatt 1973) was achieved by families that had received 9
months of Target Teaching training;

(e) achieving the product (Receptive Language gains) process (Target Teaching
strategies) relationship required a familiarisation with the teaching of receptive
language skills, which, as this research showed was not developed by parent or child in a
limited three month period. "Systems modification" as described by Zifferblatt (1973)
was to all intents and purposes non-existent in those families that received only 3
months training. This view is supported by Murray (1959) who argued that parents of
the intellectually handicapped required lifelong help. Similarly Cunningham (1977)
emphasised that parents of the intellectually handicapped are concerned with long term
objectives and sustained treatment because of the permanence and totality of their
children's learning disability.

The RRLA scores at 0_6 demonstrate that the group that received most training in the use of
Target Teaching techniques would be most likely to maintain receptive language gains. Cooper
Moodley and Reynell (1979) when writing about verbal comprehension and expressive language
gains in their Developmental Language Programme (DLP) point out that the intellectually
handicapped needed a longer time for treatment to be effective:

"We found that in two to three years these very retarded children made a language
acceleration equivalent to that made by the intellectually normal children in one year" (p.
68).

Since Cooper Moodley and Reynell (1979) used the Reynell Developmental Scales
(RDLS) to assess the receptive language (verbal comprehension) and expressive language of the
children in their five year study and expressed the gains in percentages, it is instructive to
compare their children's percentage gains, with those percentage gains of the children in this
study (see Table 5.2, 5.6, 5.7 and 5.10).

There is an indication (see Tables 5.1 and 5.2) that had the interventions for children in this
study continued beyond 9 months or indeed beyond 21 months for Groups B and C, that their
RRLA gain scores could be regarded as quite comparable with the RRLA gains achieved by the
E.S.N(S). class of the Cooper Moodley Reynell (1979) Developmental Language Programme
(DLP).

It should be noticed that children in the Language Programme only (Group D)
demonstrated very **little** improvement in RRLA scores (see Table 5.1 and 5.2). Their 5 per cent
RRLA gain over 21 months compares unfavourably with the 30 per cent RRLA gain over 5 years
of children in the Cooper Moodley Reynell (1979) "No Help Control Group". However, there
are differences between these groups that should be noted, before a comparison can be
considered valid.

These differences are:

(a) that the DLP "No Help Control Group" (N = 20) were considerably more heterogeneous in
the nature of their language handicaps. In addition there were far fewer children with "acute"
language handicaps;

(b) that there were no moderate or severely intellectually handicapped children reported in the
DLP Control Group and therefore it can be assumed that the non-verbal IQ score was
considerably higher than the mean Stanford IQ score of 39.8 SD.9.7 reported for Group D
(see Appendix VI);

(c) that the DLP Control Group parents were referred "before any help was available at the
Wolfson Centre". However, parents in Group D were aware of alternative interventions
available to other families. There was evidence that this adversely affected their motivation.

For example, two families refused to join Group D (see above p. 66). Furthermore, Roos (1975 p. 354-355) indicates that an active role for parents in intervention programmes for the intellectually handicapped enhances their feelings of self-worth, whereas no involvement or a passive role is likely to enhance parents' feelings of frustration and helplessness. The home visits in Stage 1 (see above Ch. 3, p. 55) indicated that only close and regular parent contact with professionals and the promise of follow-up visits resulted in parents carefully reading the distributed literature. Therefore the mere provision of a structured written programme without regular professional contact was observed by these parents to be "frustrating, if not depressing" with the result that " . . . hardly any teaching has taken place". In fact the mere provision of a written programme when parents were aware of other alternatives could be regarded as depressing and therefore of less help than a "no help" situation in which no alternatives existed.

Differences in Comprehension between boys and girls:

The results indicating no statistical difference in the acquisition of receptive language skills by boys and girls confirm the earlier findings of Schneider and Vallon (1954), Spreen (1965a) and Fried (1977). For example, Fried (1977) demonstrated that girls performed "a little better" than boys in verbal comprehension skills in both Down's syndrome and the undifferentiated groups of the mentally handicapped. However, in the brain damaged groups the boys performed "a little better" than the girls. Nowhere in Fried's study of 202 mentally handicapped subjects (116 boys and 86 girls, CA. 12.4 IQ 44.6) was the difference between boys and girls in measured receptive language skills statistically significant ($p < 0.05$). It should be noticed however, that experienced speech therapists such as Renfrew (1972) do make reference to the possibility of different time of onset in comprehension and speech between boys and girls. Therefore, this continues to be an issue for parents, even though, there was no difference in the ability of intellectually handicapped boys and girls to comprehend what was said.

Differences between different etiologies of intellectual handicap:

The language comprehension of Down's syndrome, Brain Damaged and other intellectually handicapped children has aroused research interest particularly since Lyle's work (Lyle 1959, 1960a, 1960b, 1961). Lyle (1959) found a significant difference of nine months verbal MA (using the verbal scores of the Minnesota Pre-School Scale of Intelligence) between Down's syndrome and non-Down's syndrome children in institutions but no significant difference between these groups in his day school sample. As indicated above (Ch. 3) all the children in this programme lived at home. The comparison of RRLA scores between different etiology groups of intellectually handicapped children over a period of 33 months confirmed the situation of "no difference between the comprehension skills of different groups of intellectually handicapped children living at home" that Lyle first noticed. Furthermore, the results presented above are of interest to parents of the intellectually handicapped because they support Lenneberg's position that the delayed comprehension and speech of Down's syndrome children, in comparison with other groups of intellectually handicapped children, has much more to do with the motivation of the Down's syndrome child than with any pathology (Lenneberg 1967 p. 309-315). In addition, Johnson and Olley (1971) point out that when Down's syndrome children were matched on IQ with brain damaged subjects and with undifferentiated retarded subjects then "few differences were found in their comprehension and none were significant".

Murphy (1956) cited by Johnson and Olley (1971) has stressed the importance of paying attention to both chronological age (CA) and mental age (MA) in any study comparing the comprehension skills of different groups of intellectually handicapped children. Slobin (1966) found a significant association of CA and comprehension in intellectually-average children but no association of comprehension skills and CA with intellectually handicapped children. Similarly Semmel and Dolley (1971) found that comprehension ability is not one which can be expected to develop with increasing CA or to be more pronounced at relatively higher IQ levels. This contrasts with the significant association of comprehension skills and CA for Down's syndrome children found by Lenneberg, Nichols and Rosenberger (1964) and replicated by

Evans and Hampson (1968). The comparison [...]
children (Mean CA 63 months) and the Mentally [...]
support the findings of Lenneberg, Nichols and Rose[...]
Herriot's evidence of developing strategies of compr[...]
(1976) write about plateaus in the comprehension and [...]
related to CA. The CA plateaus referred to by Swann [...]
of the Down's syndrome and Mentally Handicapped [...]
MANCOVA of the RRLA scores at observation poin[...]
intellectual handicap is due to no known organic origin (u[...]
O_1 and O_2 as covariates) and Down's syndrome childr[...]
positively significant difference in their RRLA scores. (F=[...]
such the RRLA scores in this comparison may be regarded a[...]
initial difference was removed, then there was no observed [...]
However, as the literature demonstrates, the comprehensi[...]
Handicapped children always seem to be superior to the D[...]
1965a Blount 1968, Johnson and Olley 1971, Fried 1977). T[...]
example at O_6 when the mean CA of the Down's syndrome gro[...]
RRLA mean scores of 36.4 months was below the RRLA mean s[...]
38.1 months when their mean CA was 8 years 2 months (see [...]

The results comparing the Receptive Language skills of [...]
intellectually handicapped children illustrate the following:

(i) that there was no significant difference in the ability to compre[...]
by the Reynell Developmental Language Scales, of Down's sy[...]
damaged children, or of an undifferentiated group of intellectu[...]
other than Down's syndrome children.

(ii) that there was a positively significant difference in the ability to c[...]
measured by the Reynell Developmental Language Scales, of Do[...]
and children whose mental handicap was due to no known organ[...]
appeared that this ability to comprehend what was said depended o[...]
comprehension strategies (see above p. 85) (and below Ch. 8) and t[...]
sion strategies (Herriot 1970) were also related to chronological age[...]
may therefore be regarded as a guide, as to whether a child was likely to[...]
of "take off", or was in fact in a "plateau period", in which few gains[...]
ability were apparent or could be expected.

Differences between children at different language levels:

Linking chronological age to measured language age provided a conve[...]
reference. Yet Lenneberg stressed that there was no physiological or biochemica[...]
particular chronological age should signal the completion of particular language [...]
the onset of new ones (Lenneberg 1967). However, what was clear in this study (se[...]
5.10 and 5.11) was that if the normal maturation function is slowed down then lan[...]
were acquired later and most important (as the evidence in Tables 5.9, 5.10 and 5.11[...]
the spacing between this acquisition of comprehension skills became more and more [...]
without altering the order of sequence. Thus the average three and a half year old inte[...]
handicapped child in Group A had a measured receptive language age of 13 months (se[...]
5.9) whereas by the time this "average intellectually handicapped child" in Group A has[...]
chronological age of 6 years 3 months his measured receptive language age had increased [...]
30 months. This represented the largest measure of receptive language gain within any grou[...]
Table 5.10). Yet this pattern of increasingly prolonged spacing between the acquisitio[...]
comprehension skills was still evident for all other groups and sub-groups (see Tables 5.9, [...]
and 5.11).

ɤ Mentally Handicapped: Children whose intellectual handicap was due to no known organic origin.

TABLE 5.12

Reynell Expressive Language Age (RELA) Estimated* and Adjusted$^{\phi}$ Mean Scores for Different Treatment Groups

Group	N	Pre-test mean O_1	Pre-test mean O_2	Post-test mean O_3	Adjusted Post-test mean O_3	Post-test mean O_4	Adjusted Post-test mean O_4	Post-test mean O_5	Adjusted Post-test mean O_5	Post-test mean O_6	Adjusted Post-test mean O_6
A	25	21.02	22.1	29.4	32.1	29.6	32.1	30.6	33.5	34.8	37.5
B	24	19.28	22.5	23.8	26.9	24.3	27.2	31.3	34.4	31.2	34.2
C	25	18.25	18.4	21.3	28.4	21.9	28.3	24.5	31.8	25.7	32.5
D	28	16.87	20.8	21.6	27.2	22.3	27.4	25.7	31.3	28.4	33.8

* Estimated mean RELA scores based on a MANOVA analysis of observed scores at observation points O_1 to O_6 inclusive.

ϕ Adjusted mean RELA scores at observation points O_3, O_4, O_5 and O_6 based on a MANCOVA analysis using pre-test RELA scores at observation points O_1 and O_2 as covariates.

FIG. 5.2

Graphical Representation of Mean Reynell Expressive Language Age Scores
& Adjusted Post-Test Scores for Treatment Groups

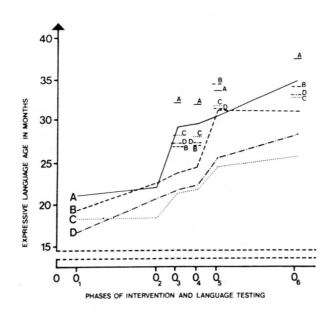

ADJUSTED SCORES

```
———————— A   Target Teaching Group A
------------- B   Social Work/Supportive Counselling Group B
.............. C   Speech Therapy Group C
-·--·--·-- D   Language Programme Only Group D
```

Yet, Jeffree & McConkey (1976a) reported that there are few studies which set out to compare the effectiveness of different interventions from the specific point of view of teaching and assessing expressive language. Rather, proponents of particular methods of teaching expressive language skills seek to demonstrate the effectiveness of their particular methods. For example, Kazdin (1979) points out that operant techniques have been widely applied to retarded and learning disabled children, particularly in relation to their developing language. Schneider and Vallon (1954 and 1955) and Hume (1978) demonstrated the improvements in the vocalisation and speech of the retarded that can occur as a result of speech therapy.

The expressive language results presented below examine the effectiveness of different interventions, the effects of sex and different etiologies on children's expressive language development, and the effects of children's stage or level of expressive language upon the success of interventions.

Comparison of Treatment Groups

1. Group A vs. Group B

Children in the experimental Target Teaching Group A (see Fig. 5.2 and Tables 5.12, 5.13 and 5.14) showed a greater improvement than children in the Social Work/Supportive Counselling Group B over the period of intervention 0_2 to 0_3 and 0_2 to 0_6 (see Fig. 3.1).

TABLE 5.13

Percentage R E L A Mean Scores ϕ Gain for Each Treatment Group During Successive Phases of Intervention

Group	% Gain 0_2 to 0_3	% Gain 0_3 to 0_4	% Gain 0_4 to 0_5	% Gain 0_5 to 0_6	% Gain 0_2 to 0_6
A	33.0	1.0	3.0	14.0	56.0
B	5.0	2.0	28.0	-	38.0
C	16.0	3.0	12.0	5.0	40.0
D	4.0	3.0	15.0	10.0	36.0

ϕ Percentage gains based on estimated R E L A mean scores. Estimated mean scores calculated by using a MANOVA of the R E L A observed scores for the period 0_1 to 0_6.

Multivariate analysis of covariance (MANCOVA) of RELA scores at observation points 0_3, 0_4, 0_5 and 0_6 indicated that the difference between the mean Reynell Expressive Language Age Scores for children in Group A and Group B was statistically significant (F=3.416, df=4 and 40.0 p<0.017). Examination of RELA mean scores at the end of each period of intervention revealed that the gains achieved by both Groups was greatest during the first period of the structured Target Teaching 0_2 to 0_3 for Group A and 0_4 to 0_5 for Group B (see Table 5.12 and 5.13). Examination of the step down F tests (see Table 5.14) revealed that it was at the end of Phase 1_1 at 0_3, that the most significant difference between RELA scores appeared and, that there was a statistically significant difference between the adjusted RELA scores of the experimental Target Teaching Group A and the Social Work/Supportive Counselling Group B at the 0.05 level of significance (step down F=10.256 p<0.003).

2. Group A vs. Group C

Children in the experimental Target Teaching Group A (see Fig. 5.2 and Tables 5.12 and 5.13) showed a greater improvement in RELA scores over the period of intervention 0_2 to 0_3 and 0_2 and 0_6 than children in the Speech Therapy Group C (see Table 5.13). However, multivariate

TABLE 5.14

Probability Levels for Univariate and Step Down F Values When R E L A
Mean Scores for Groups A and B were Compared ∮ at Observation Points
0_3, 0_4, 0_5 and 0_6.

Variable	Error Mean Square	Hypothesis Mean Square	Univariate F	P Less Than	Step Down F	P Less Than
RELA 0_3	11.592	118.89	10.256	0.003	10.256	0.003
RELA 0_4	18.956	115.97	6.118	0.018	0.003	0.959
RELA 0_5	110.875	75.61	0.682	0.414	3.313	0.076
RELA 0_6	49.588	0.32	0.007	0.936	0.089	0.768

∮ Based on MANCOVA with pretests R E L A at observation points 0_1 and
0_2 as covariates.

R E L A: Reynell Expressive Language Age.

analysis of covariance (MANCOVA) of RELA scores at observation points 0_3, 0_4, 0_5 and 0_6
revealed that the difference between the mean Reynell Expressive Language Age scores for
children in Group A and Group C was not statistically significant (F=0.286 df=4 and 40.0
p<0.886). Likewise the difference between the mean RELA scores for children in Group A and
Group C at observation points 0_3 and 0_4 was not statistically significant (see Table 5.15).

TABLE 5.15

Probability Levels for Univariate and Step Down F Values when
R E L A Mean Scores for Groups A and C were Compared ∮ at Observation
Points 0_3 and 0_4.

Variable	Error Mean Square	Hypothesis Mean Square	Univariate F	P Less Than	Step Down F	P Less Than
RELA 0_3	11.592	2.68	0.2315	0.633	0.2315	0.633
RELA 0_4	18.956	7.43	0.3917	0.535	0.1558	0.695

∮ Based on MANCOVA with pre-tests R E L A at observation points 0_1 and
0_2 as covariates.
R E L A: Reynell Expressive Language Age.

3. Group A vs. Group D

Children in the experimental Target Teaching Group A (see Fig. 5.2 and Tables 5.12 and
5.13) showed a greater improvement in RELA scores over the period of intervention 0_2 to 0_3 and
0_2 to 0_6 (see Tables 5.12 and 5.13) than children in the Language Programme only Group D.
Multivariate analysis of covariance (MANCOVA) of RELA scores at observation points 0_3,

0_4, 0_5 and 0_6 indicated that the difference between the mean Reynell Expressive Language Age Scores for children in Group A and Group B was statistically significant ($F=3.032$, df=4 and 40. p<0.028). Examination of the step-down F tests (see Table 5.16) indicated that it was at the end of Phase I at 0_3, that the most relevant subset of RELA scores appeared and that there was a statistically significant difference, between the adjusted mean RELA scores of the experimental Target Teaching Group A and the Language Programme only Group D.

TABLE 5.16

Probability Levels for Univariate and Step Down F Values when R E L A Mean Scores for Groups A and D were Compared ∅ at Observation Points 0_3, 0_4, 0_5 and 0_6.

Variable	Error Mean Square	Hypothesis Mean Square	Univariate F	P Less Than	Step Down F	P Less Than
RELA 0_3	11.592	133.24	11.49	0.002	11.49	0.002
RELA 0_4	18.956	126.61	6.68	0.013	0.011	0.920
RELA 0_5	110.875	7.87	0.07	0.791	0.690	0.411
RELA 0_6	49.588	80.73	1.63	0.210	0.441	0.510

∅ Based on MANCOVA with pre-tests R E L A at observation points 0_1 and 0_2 as covariates.
R E L A: Reynell Expressive Language Age.

4. Comparison of Boys and Girls Expressive Language Age Scores

Boys showed a greater improvement in mean RELA scores overall (0_1 to 0_6) and over the period of the intervention 0_2 to 0_6 (see Table 5.17). Girls showed a greater improvement in mean RELA scores over the period of the intervention 0_2 to 0_5. However, multivariate analysis of variance (MANOVA) of the RELA scores at observation points 0_1, 0_2, 0_3, 0_4, 0_5 and 0_6 revealed that the differences between the mean Reynell Expressive Language Age Scores for Boys and Girls was not statistically significant ($F=1.91$, df=6 and 40 p<0.103).

Comparison of Etiology Groups. Expressive Language Age Scores.

5. Down's Syndrome Children vs. All Other Intellectually Handicapped Children.

Which group of children showed a greater improvement depended on the time period examined (see Table 5.18). Over the total period of the programme 0_1 to 0_6 the Down's syndrome children demonstrated greatest improvement though their greatest gain took place in the first year 0_1 to 0_2 and thereafter all other intellectually handicapped children demonstrated a slightly greater improvement in RELA mean scores. However, multivariate analysis of variance (MANOVA) of RELA scores at observation points 0_1, 0_2, 0_3, 0_4, 0_5 and 0_6 indicated that the difference between the mean Reynell Expressive Language Age scores for Down's syndrome children and all other intellectually handicapped children was not statistically significant ($F=1.676$, df=6 and 40.0 p<0.152).

6. Down's Syndrome Children vs. Brain Damaged Children

The Brain Damaged group showed a slightly greater improvement in RELA scores than the Down's syndrome children (see Table 5.18). However, multivariate analysis of variance

107

TABLE 5.17

Mean Reynell Expressive Language Age (RELA) Scores in Months for Boys and Girls at Observation Points O_1 to O_6 Inclusive and Percentage Gains^φ in RELA Scores in Each Time Period

Group	N	CA at O_1 mths.	RELA at O_1	RELA at O_2	% Gain O_1 to O_2	RELA at O_3	% Gain O_2 to O_3	RELA at O_4	% Gain O_3 to O_4	RELA at O_5	% Gain O_4 to O_5	RELA at O_6	% Gain O_5 to O_6	% Gain O_1 to O_6	% Gain O_2 to O_5
All Boys	58	72	22.8	25.2	10.5	27.6	9.5	28.5	3.0	32.1	13.0	35.7	11.0	56.0	27.0
All Girls	44	62	22.3	24.2	8.5	27.6	14.0	27.4	-	32.3	18.0	31.6	-2.0	42.0	33.0

φ Estimated mean RELA scores based on a MANOVA of the observed RELA mean scores at observation points O_1, O_2, O_3, O_4, O_5 and O_6.

TABLE 5.18

Mean Reynell Expressive Language Age Scores$^{\emptyset}$ in Months for Different Etiology Groups at Observation Points O_1 to O_6 and Percentage Gains in RELA Scores in Each Time Period

Group	N	C.A. at O_1 mths	RELA at O_1	RELA at O_2	% Gain O_1 to O_2	RELA at O_3	% Gain O_2 to O_3	RELA at O_4	% Gain O_3 to O_4	RELA at O_5	% Gain O_4 to O_5	RELA at O_6	% Gain O_5 to O_6	% Gain O_1 to O_6	% Gain O_2 to O_6
Down's Syndrome	57	63	20.9	24.3	16.3	26.8	10.3	27.6	3.0	31.3	13.4	32.5	3.8	55.5	33.7
All Other I.H. Children	45	72	23.8	25.0	5.0	28.2	12.8	28.3	-	33.0	16.6	34.5	4.5	45.0	38.0
Brain Damaged	16	75	21.5	24.6	14.4	24.7	-	25.2	2.0	31.5	25.0	34.1	8.3	58.6	38.6
Mentally Handi-capped	10	98	27.2	30.1	10.7	33.0	9.6	33.4	1.2	34.2	2.4	37.3	9.1	37.1	24.0

$^{\emptyset}$ Estimated mean RELA scores based on a MANOVA analysis of the observed RELA scores observation points O_1, O_2, O_3, O_4, O_5 and O_6.

(MANOVA of RELA scores at observation points O_1, O_2, O_3, O_4, O_5 and O_6 indicated that the difference between the mean Reynell Expressive Language Age scores for Down's syndrome children and children classified as Brain Damaged was not statistically significant ($F=1.604$, df$=6$ and 40.0 p<0.171).

7. Down's Syndrome Children vs. Mentally Handicapped Children ∅

Down's Syndrome children showed greater improvement in RELA scores than children whose intellectual handicap was due to no known organic origin. However, multivariate analysis of variance (MANOVA) of RELA scores at observation points O_1, O_2, O_3, O_4, O_5 and O_6 revealed that the difference between the mean RELA scores for the two groups was not statistically significant ($F=2.324$, df$=6$ and 40.0 p<0.0511). The difference of 6.3 months (see Table 5.18) between the mean RELA scores of Down's syndrome children at O_1 (mean RELA scores $=$ 20.9 months) and children whose intellectual handicap was due to no known organic origin (mean RELA score $=$ 27.2 months) accounted for the greatest amount of variance of the MANOVA analysis O_1 to O_6 (step down F at O_1 $=12.63$ p<0.0001). However, a MANOVA of the RELA scores at observation points O_3, O_4, O_5 and O_6 indicated that the difference between the groups was also not statistically significant ($F=1.082$, df$=4$ and 42 p<0.378).

Comparison of Language Levels Within Treatment Groups: Expressive Language Age Scores.

8. Experimental Target Teaching Group A. Level 1 vs. Levels 2 & 3

The advantage in mean RELA gain scores as indicated by per centage RELA gains at each successive time interval favoured children at level 1 (CA 3 years 6 months at O_1) (see also Tables 5.19 and 5.20). The difference between the mean RELA scores of children at different language levels was statistically significant. For example, a MANOVA of the RELA scores at observation points O_1, O_2, O_3, O_4, O_5 and O_6 indicated that the difference between the groups was statistically significant ($F=35.02$, df$=6$ and 40.0 p<0.0001). Similarly a MANOVA of the mean RELA scores at observation points O_3, O_4, O_5 and O_6 indicated that the difference between the mean RELA scores for children at different language levels was also statistically significant ($F=13.842$, df$=4$ and 42 p<0.0001). However, a multivariate analysis of covariance (MANCOVA) of RELA scores at observation points O_3, O_4, O_5 and O_6 using the RELA pre-test scores at O_1 and O_2 as covariates, indicated that the difference in mean RELA scores for children at different language levels was also statistically significant at the 0.05 level of significance ($F=3.148$, df$=4$ and 40.0 p<0.024) with the direction in favour of children at language level 1.

9. Social Work/Supportive Counselling Group B. Level 1 vs. Levels 2 & 3

The advantage in mean RELA gain scores as indicated by per centage RELA gains at each successive time interval generally favoured children at language level 1 (see Table 5.20). However, at intervals O_1 to O_2 (gains of 18.2 per cent for levels 2 and 3 compared with 11.5 per cent for level 1) and O_4 to O_5 (gains of 32.0 per cent for levels 2 and 3 compared with 20.3 per cent for level 1) the advantage in RELA gain scores favoured children at language levels 2 and 3 (CA 7 years 1 month at O_1). The difference between the mean RELA scores of children at different language levels was statistically significant. For example, a MANOVA of the RELA scores at observation points O_1, O_2, O_3, O_4, O_5 and O_6 indicated that the difference between the two language levels was statistically significant ($F=23.851$, df$=6$ and p<0.0001). Similarly a MANOVA of the mean RELA scores at observation points O_3, O_4, O_5 and O_6 inclusive (after the Social Work/Supportive Counselling Target Teaching Intervention) indicated that the difference between the mean RELA scores of the different language levels was also statistically significant ($F=10.723$ df$=4$ and 42 p<0.0001). However, a MANCOVA of the RELA scores at observation points O_3, O_4, O_5 and O_6 using the RELA pre-test scores at O_1 and O_2 as covariates indicated that the difference in mean RELA scores for children at different language levels was not statistically significant ($F=2.395$ df$=4$ and 40.0 p<0.067).

∅ Mentally Handicapped children: Children whose intellectual handicap is due to no known organic origin.

110

TABLE 5.19

Reynell Expressive Language Age Mean Scoresϕ at Observation points O_1 to O_6 for Language Levels within Treatment Groups

Group	Language Level	N	Mean CA at O_1 in Months	SD in Months	O_1 RELA	O_2 RELA	O_3 RELA	O_4 RELA	O_5 RELA	O_6 RELA
A	1	12	42	17.8	8.6	10.3	18.9	19.3	18.9	25.0
	2 & 3	13	80	28.5	33.5	34.0	39.8	39.9	42.3	44.6
B	1	12	57	30.0	7.8	8.7	11.6	13.3	16.0	16.5
	2 & 3	12	85	34.8	30.8	36.4	36.0	35.3	46.6	45.8
C	1	13	45	15.4	6.5	9.2	10.4	11.5	12.5	14.4
	2 & 3	12	97	31.6	30.0	27.6	32.3	32.3	36.5	37.1
D	1	13	51	11.3	8.2	11.6	12.2	13.0	14.3	20.7
	2 & 3	15	84	28.7	25.6	30.0	31.0	31.6	37.2	36.2

ϕ Estimated mean RELA scores obtained using a MANOVA of the observed RELA mean scores O_1 to O_6 inclusive.

Language Level 1 refers to children whose combined mean Reynell Developmental Language Age (RDLA) score at O_1 was 18 months or less.

Language Levels 2 and 3 refer to children whose combined RDLA score at O_1 was greater than 18 months.

TABLE 5.20

Per Centage R E L A Age Gains for Language Levels Within Treatment Groups Following Each Period of Intervention

GROUP	Language Level	N	% Gain O_1 to O_2	% Gain O_2 to O_3	% Gain O_3 to O_4	% Gain O_4 to O_5	% Gain O_5 to O_6	% Gain O_1 to O_6	% Gain O_2 to O_6
A	1	12	20.0	83.5	2.0	-2.0	32.3	190.7	142.7
	2 & 3	13	1.5	17.1	-	6.0	5.4	33.1	31.2
B	1	12	11.5	33.3	14.7	20.3	3.1	111.5	89.7
	2 & 3	12	18.2	-1.0	-2.0	32.0	-1.7	48.7	25.8
C	1	13	41.5	13.0	10.6	8.7	15.2	121.5	56.5
	2 & 3	12	-8.0	17.0	-	13.0	1.6	23.7	34.4
D	1	13	41.5	5.2	6.6	10.0	44.8	152.4	78.4
	2 & 3	15	17.2	3.3	2.0	17.7	-2.7	41.4	20.7

Per centage gains calculated from estimated mean R E L A scores

Estimated mean R E L A scores based on a MANOVA analysis of the observed R E L A scores O_1 to O_6 inclusive.

Language Level 1 refers to children whose combined mean R D L A score at O_1 was 18 months or less.

Language Levels 2 & 3 refer to children whose combined mean R D L A score at O_1 was greater than 18 months.

10. Speech Therapy Group C. Level 1 vs. Levels 2 & 3

The advantage in RELA gain scores, as indicated by per centage RELA gains at each successive time interval, generally favoured children at language level 1 (CA 3 years 9 months at O_1) (see Tables 5.19, 5.20 and 5.21). However, at intervals O_2 to O_3 (a gain of 17.0 per cent for levels 2 and 3 compared with 13.0 per cent for level 1) and O_4 to O_5 (a gain of 13.0 per cent for levels 2 and 3 compared with 8.7 per cent for level 1) the advantage in RELA gain scores slightly favoured children at language levels 2 and 3 (CA of 8 years 1 month at O_1). The difference between the mean RELA scores of children at different language levels was statistically significant. For example, a MANOVA of the mean RELA scores at observation points O_1, O_2, O_3, O_4, O_5 and O_6 indicated that the difference between the two language levels was statistically significant (F=21.376 df=6 and 40.0 p<0.0001). Similarly a MANOVA of the mean RELA scores at observation points O_3, O_4, O_5 and O_6 (after the Speech Therapy, Target Teaching intervention) indicated that the difference between the mean RELA scores of children at the two different language levels was also statistically significant (F=7.80, df=4 and 42.0 p<0.0001). However, a MANCOVA of the RELA scores at observation points O_3, O_4, O_5 and O_6 using the RELA pre-test scores at observation points O_1 and O_2 as covariates indicated that the difference in mean RELA scores for children at the two different language levels was not statistically significant (F=0.473, df=4 and 40 p<0.755).

11. Language Programme Only Group D. Level 1 vs. Levels 2 & 3.

The advantage in RELA gain scores as indicated by per centage RELA gains at each successive time interval generally favoured children at language level 1 (CA 4 years 3 months at O_1) (see Tables 5.19, 5.20 and 5.21). However, at interval O_4 to O_5 (a gain of 17.7 per cent for children at language levels 2 and 3 compared with 10.0 per cent for children at level 1) the advantage in RELA gain scores slightly favoured children at language levels 2 and 3 (CA of 7 years at O_1). The difference between the mean RELA scores of children at different language levels was statistically significant as indicated by a MANOVA of those RELA scores. For example, a MANOVA of the mean RELA scores at observation points O_1, O_2, O_3, O_4, O_5 and O_6 indicated that the difference between the two language levels was statistically significant (F=15.388 df=6 and 40.0 p<0.0001). Similarly, a MANOVA of the RELA scores at observation points O_3, O_4, O_5 and O_6 indicated that the difference between the mean RELA scores of children at the two different language levels was statistically significant (F=7.399 df=4 and 42.0 p<0.0002). However, a MANCOVA of RELA scores at observation points O_3, O_4, O_5 and O_6 using the RELA pre-test scores at O_1 and O_2 as covariates indicted that the difference in mean RELA scores for children at the two different language levels was not statistically significant (F=1.798, df=4 and 40.0 p<0.148).

Discussion of Expressive Language Results

Nine months of applying a structured Target Teaching programme was more effective in improving the expressive language skills of intellectually handicapped children than either, a Social Work/Supportive Counselling intervention plus three months of Target Teaching, or an intervention which provided parents with only the written Language Programme. The results in this study do contrast with Heifetz's finding that there was no significant difference in the language development of the intellectually handicapped no matter whether their families were provided with the written programme only, or with the written programme and back-up support in the form of telephone consultations, training groups and home visits (Heifetz 1977). In this study the superiority of the structured Target Teaching programme over the Social Work/Supportive Counselling intervention or the Language Programme only intervention was noticeable in both the first three months of intervention and in the following eighteen months.

However, nine months of structured Target Teaching was not significantly more effective in improving the expressive language skills of the intellectually handicapped than six months of developmental Speech Therapy plus three months of Target Teaching. Furthermore Target Teaching was not superior to Speech Therapy during the three month or six month period. It would therefore, be an over-simplification, to claim the superiority of positive reinforcement teaching techniques in developing the spontaneous utterances, single syllable sounds and words,

TABLE 5.21

Reynell Expressive Language Age Adjusted ∅ Mean Scores at Observation Points O_3, O_4, O_5 and O_6 for Language Levels Within Treatment Groups Following each Period of Intervention

GROUP	Language Level	N	Adj. R E L A at O_3	Adj. R E L A at O_4	Adj. R E L A at O_5	Adj. R E L A at O_6
A	1	12	36.9	35.6	37.2	42.4
	2 & 3	13	27.4	28.6	29.8	32.6
B	1	12	31.2	31.1	36.0	35.5
	2 & 3	12	22.2	23.3	32.9	33.0
C	1	13	30.2	29.4	32.5	33.5
	2 & 3	12	26.6	27.2	31.0	31.6
D	1	13	29.2	28.4	31.4	37.1
	2 & 3	15	25.2	26.4	31.2	30.6

∅ Adjusted mean R E L A scores O_3 to O_6 based on a MANCOVA analysis of R E L A scores at observation points O_3, O_4, O_5 and O_6 using pre-test observed R E L A scores at O_1 and O_2 as covariates.

Language Level 1 refers to children whose combined mean R D L A score at O_1 was 18 months or less.

Language Levels 2 & 3 refer to children whose combined mean R D L A score at O_1 was greater than 18 months.

or word combinations and simple sentences of the intellectually handicapped despite the fact that the advantages in expressive language gain scores was with the Target Teaching group.

Hume (1978) described the improvements in vocalisation and meaningful speech production of children in the Speech Therapy group. This description was well supported by their expressive language results. The speech therapists in this programme demonstrated their skill in getting children to produce speech sounds, words and meaningful word order. The results of this programme demonstrated, that, a combination of the sequencing and developmental skills of the speech therapist, allied to the shaping and positive reinforcement procedures of operant teaching techniques, would provide, the most effective means of both teaching children expressive language skills and of providing relevant parent training. This combination, or integration of techniques, is necessary, in order to avoid the confusion that occurs for parents, when they are presented with contrasting teaching techniques.

There are few studies that have undertaken such a long term intervention (Bronfenbrenner 1974). The results in this programme confirm other findings (Cooper Moodley and Reynell 1979; Lovaas, Koegel, Simmons and Long 1973), that the longer the period of intervention, particularly where positive reinforcement techniques have been applied, the greater is the likelihood of achieving improvement in children's expressive language. However, it should also be noted that the maximum gains by the intellectually handicapped children appeared in the first three months of the structured Target Teaching programme (time period 0_2 to 0_3 for Group A and time period 0_4 to 0_5 for Group B) and thereafter the gains were not maintained at that rate of improvement.

Careful examination of the expressive language results indicated that boys do not do better than girls, or vice versa. These results also confirm Fried's findings that there was no significant difference in the measured speech production and intelligibility of boys and girls (Fried 1977). However, discussions with parents throughout this programme, still indicate that they are likely to go on questioning the likelihood of differences in the ability of their intellectually handicapped sons, or daughters, to acquire meaningful speech.

Much research has been undertaken comparing the expressive language skills of different etiology groups of intellectually handicapped children (Bijou 1944 and 1945, Erwin 1961, Fried 1977, Guda and Griffith 1962, Papania 1954, Sievers 1959, Spradlin 1963a and 1963b, Spreen 1965a and 1965b Wolfe 1950). The results of this "Parents as Language Therapists" study demonstrated that there was no statistically significant difference between the expressive language skills of Down's syndrome children and all other intellectually handicapped children. It should be noted however, that much attention was given to motivation for the Down's syndrome children (as recommended by Lenneberg 1967). It is believed that this accounted for the comparably better expressive language performance of the Down's syndrome children in this study than that noted by Johnson and Olley (1971) or by Lyle (1959).

There was no statistically significant difference in the measured expressive language performance of Brain Damaged and Down's syndrome children, although, the advantage in expressive language gain scores was with the brain damaged children. Speech therapists' assessment (Hume 1978) was that the brain damaged children "tended to do better than the Down's syndrome children on both verbal imitation and speech production". This finding is similar to that which appears in Gallagher's comprehensive study comparing the language performance of brain injured and non-brain injured mentally retarded children (Gallagher 1957).

Comparison of the speech production ability of Down's syndrome children and familial retards often provides conflicting results (Blount 1968, Fried 1977). In this study there was no statistical difference between the expressive language skills of Down's syndrome and children whose mental handicap was due to no known organic origin, especially when chronological ages were comparable. The advantage in expressive language gains slightly favoured the Down's syndrome children. However, careful attention in particular was given to motivation in the teaching of expressive language skills to the Down's syndrome children. Both parents and teachers pointed out that this enhanced both the Down's syndrome children's "self concept and social competence". This in turn had the effect, of encouraging both parents and their Down's syndrome children, to persist with rehearsing expressive language tasks. This finding, of the effects of improved expressed language development on self concept and social competence and vice versa, is similar to that reported by Harvey, Yep and Sellin (1966).

Younger children, at a lower expressive language age level, demonstrated greater improvement in expressive language age scores than older children who commenced the programme at a higher expressive language age level. However, the difference between the expressive language age scores following the different interventions was not statistically significant, except in the case of children experiencing the structured Target Teaching programme. In the Target Teaching group there was a statistically significant difference in the expressive language age scores of the younger children, at the lower expressive language age level, when compared with the expressive language age scores of the older children, at the higher expressive language age level. The greatest improvement in expressive language age scores, was achieved by the younger children, who commenced the programme at the lower expressive language age level. It appeared therefore, that structured teaching over an extended period was more effective in improving the measured expressive language of younger children (who, when the intervention commenced, were at the level of reflexive sound production and at the level of production of some understandable sounds and words), than in improving the measured expressive language of older children, (who were required to learn increasingly complicated skills, such as accurate reproduction of words, increasing vocabulary and, if possible, two word and simple sentence production). However, a plateau effect was noted for both groups in the rate of improvement in measured expressive language. It would seem therefore, that only a structured teaching programme applied over many years could provide the information of just how long this plateau feature lasts and, when the next take off could be expected. Fay and Butler (1968) have indicated how expressive language skills acquired at a lower level, form the basis for **later** expressive language development. A structured teaching programme, which can take account of both the expressive language plateau feature and the fact that skills acquired at a lower level form the basis for higher order expressive language skills, may, if applied over a long enough period, result in the acquisition of more automatic meaningful speech. The evidence from this programme demonstrated that this was a possibility.

The theoretical framework underlying this "Parents as Language Therapists" teaching programme emphasised the role of a hierarchy of expressive language processes. These processes took account of both comprehension skills and speech production. The teaching programme aimed to both improve measured expressive language performance and also, to strengthen those expressive language skills, on which future improvement depended. This was necessary because the study demonstrated the children's deficiencies in expressive language skills. These basic deficiencies greatly impeded the children's expressive language development.

Whether the structured teaching in turn could result in higher and higher levels of expressive language skills depends not only on the children in the programme, but, on the length of time during which structured teaching is applied, and also, on the attention given to precision and functionality. Teaching programmes designed to improve these children's expressive language skills have to be skill specific rather than global.

TESTING OF HYPOTHESES

The purpose of the computations was to use statistical inferential tests to decide whether the data supported the hypotheses concerning the main effects of the factors treatment, sex, etiology and language level. Using the multivariate analysis of covariance (MANCOVA) or the multivariate analysis of variance (MANOVA) the mean RRLA or RELA scores determined the acceptance or rejection of the hypotheses.

The acceptance or rejection of the hypotheses are presented below. **The Hypotheses.** Eight Sets of Hypotheses are listed:

HYPOTHESES FOR RECEPTIVE LANGUAGE TESTS

1. **Treatment Group Comparisons: Receptive Language Age Scores.**
   Hypothesis Ia That children in the Target Teaching Group A perform differently on the Reynell Receptive Language Age Test at observation points O_3, O_4, O_5 and O_6 from children in the Social Work/Supportive Counselling Group B, is rejected. There was no significant difference in their performance (see above p. 88).
   Hypothesis Ib That children in the Target Teaching Group A perform differently on the Reynell Receptive Language Age Test at observation points O_3 and O_4 from children in the Social Work/Supportive Counselling Group B, is rejected. There was no significant difference in their performance (see above p. 88).
   Hypothesis Ic That children in the Target Teaching Group A perform differently on the Reynell Receptive Language Age Test at observation points O_3, O_4, O_5 and O_6 from children in the Speech Therapy Group C, is rejected. There was no significant difference in their performance (see above p. 89).
   Hypothesis Id That children in the Target Teaching Group A perform differently on the Reynell Receptive Language Age Test at observation points O_3 and O_4 from children in the Speech Therapy Group C, is rejected. There was no significant difference in their performance (see above p. 89).
   Hypothesis Ie That children in the Target Teaching Group A perform differently on the Reynell Receptive Language Age Test at observation points O_3, O_4, O_5 and O_6 from children in the Language Programme only Group D, is accepted. Children in Target Teaching Group A perform significantly better ($p<0.0003$) than children in the Language Programme only Group D (see above p. 89).
   Hypothesis If That children in the Target Teaching Group A perform differently on the Reynell Receptive Language Age Test at observation points O_3 and O_4 from children in the Language Programme only Group D, is accepted at observation point O_3. Children in Target Teaching Group A perform significantly better ($p<0.0001$) than children in the Language Programme only Group D (see above p. 90).

2. **Boys and Girls Comparisons: Receptive Language Age Scores.**
   Hypothesis IIa That all intellectually handicapped boys perform differently on the Reynell Receptive Language Age Test at observation points O_1, O_2, O_3, O_4, O_5 and O_6 from all intellectually handicapped girls, is rejected. There was no significant difference in their performance (see above p. 90).

3. **Etiology Group Comparisons: Receptive Language Age Scores.**
   Hypothesis IIIa That all Down's syndrome children perform differently on the Reynell Receptive Language Age Test at observation points O_1, O_2, O_3, O_4, O_5 and O_6 from all other intellectually handicapped children, is rejected. There was no significant difference in their performance (see above p. 90).
   Hypothesis IIIb That all Down's syndrome children perform differently on the Reynell Receptive Language Age Test at observation points O_1, O_2, O_3, O_4, O_5 and O_6 from all children classified as Brain Damaged, is rejected. There was no significant difference in their performance (see above p. 90).
   Hypothesis IIIc That all Down's syndrome children perform differently on the Reynell Receptive Language Age Test at observation points O_1, O_2, O_3, O_4, O_5 and O_6 from children whose intellectual handicap is due to no known organic origin, is accepted. Down's syndrome children do not perform as well as Mentally Handicapped children whose handicap is due to no known organic origin ($p<0.009$) (see above p. 90).

4. **Language Levels Comparison: Receptive Language Age Scores.**
Hypothesis IVa That children at Language Level 1 in Target Teaching Group A perform differently on the Reynell Receptive Language Age Test at observation points $0_3, 0_4, 0_5$ and 0_6 from children at Language Levels 2 and 3 in Target Teaching Group A is rejected. There was no significant difference in their performance (see above p. 93).

Hypothesis IVb That children at Language Level 1 in Social Work/Supportive Counselling Group B perform differently on the Reynell Receptive Language Age Test at observation points 0_3, 0_4, 0_5 and 0_6 from children at Language Levels 2 and 3 in Social Work/Supportive Counselling Group B is rejected. There was no significant difference in their performance (see above p. 97).

Hypothesis IVc That children at Language Level 1 in the Speech Therapy Group C perform differently on the Reynell Receptive Language Age Test at observation points $0_3, 0_4, 0_5$ and 0_6 from children at Language Levels 2 and 3 in the Speech Therapy Group C is rejected. There was no significant difference in their performance (see above p. 97).

Hypothesis IVd That children at Language Level 1 in the Language Programme only Group D perform differently on the Reynell Receptive Language Age Test at observation points 0_3, 0_4, 0_5 and 0_6 from children at Language Levels 2 and 3 in the Language Programme only Group D is rejected. There was no significant difference in their performance (see above p. 97).

HYPOTHESES FOR EXPRESSIVE LANGUAGE TESTS

5. **Treatment Group Comparisons: Expressive Language Age Scores.**
Hypothesis Va That children in Target Teaching Group A perform differently on the Reynell Expressive Language Age Test at observation points 0_3, 0_4, 0_5 and 0_6 from children in the Social Work/Supportive Counselling Group B is accepted. Children in Target Teaching Goup A performed significantly better ($p<0.017$) than children in the Social Work/Supportive Counselling Group B (see above p. 105).

Hypothesis Vb That children in Target Teaching Group A perform differently on the Reynell Expressive Language Age Test at observation points 0_3 and 0_4 from children in the Social Work/Supportive Counselling Group B is accepted at observation point 0_3. Children in Target Teaching Group A performed significantly better ($p<0.003$) than children in the Social Work/Supportive Counselling Group B (see above p. 105).

Hypothesis Vc That children in Target Teaching Group A perform differently on the Reynell Expressive Language Age Test at observation points 0_3, 0_4, 0_5 and 0_6 from children in the Speech Therapy Group C is rejected. There was no significant difference in their performance (see above p. 105).

Hypothesis Vd That children in Target Teaching Group A perform differently on the Reynell Expressive Language Age Test at observation points 0_3 and 0_4 from children in the Speech Therapy Group C is rejected. There was no significant difference in their performance (see above p. 106).

Hypothesis Ve That children in the Target Teaching Group A perform differently on the Reynell Expressive Language Age Test at observation points 0_3, 0_4, 0_5 and 0_6 from children in the Language Programme only Group D is accepted. Children in Target Teaching Group A performed significantly better ($p<0.028$) than children in the Language Programme only Group D (see above p. 107).

Hypothesis Vf That children in the Target Teaching Group A perform differently on the Reynell Expressive Language Age Test at observation points 0_3 and 0_4 from children in the Language Programme only Group D is accepted at observation point 0_3. Children in Target Teaching Group A perform significantly better ($p<0.002$) than children in the Language Programme only Group D (see above p. 107).

6. **Boys and Girls Comparisons: Expressive Language Age Scores.**
Hypothesis VI That all intellectually handicapped boys perform differently on the Reynell

Expressive Language Age Test at observation points O_1, O_2, O_3, O_4, O_5 and O_6 than all intellectually handicapped girls is rejected. There was no significant difference in their performance (see above p. 107).

7. **Etiology Group Comparisons: Expressive Language Age Scores.**
   Hypothesis VIIa That all Down's Syndrome children perform differently on the Reynell Expressive Language Age Test at observation points O_1, O_2, O_3, O_4, O_5 and O_6 from all other intellectually handicapped children is rejected. There was no significant difference in their performance (see above p. 107).
   Hypothesis VIIb That all Down's Syndrome children perform differently on the Reynell Expressive Language Age Test at observation points O_1, O_2, O_3, O_4, O_5 and O_6 from all children classified as Brain Damaged is rejected. There was no significant difference in their performance (see above p. 107).
   Hypothesis VIIc That all Down's Syndrome children perform differently on the Reynell Expressive Language Age Test at observation points O_1, O_2, O_3, O_4, O_5 and O_6 from children whose intellectual handicap is due to no known organic origin is rejected. There was no significant difference in their performance (see above p. 110).

8. **Language Levels Comparisons: Expressive Language Age Scores.**
   Hypothesis VIIIa That children at Language Level 1, in Target Teaching Group A perform differently on the Reynell Expressive Language Age Test at observation points O_3, O_4, O_5 and O_6 from children at Language Levels 2 and 3 in Target Teaching Group A is accepted. Children at Language Level 1 performed significantly better ($p < 0.024$) than children at Language Levels 2 and 3 (see above p. 110).
   Hypothesis VIIIb That children at Language Level 1 in the Social Work/Supportive Counselling Group B perform differently on the Reynell Expressive Language Age Test at observation points O_3, O_4, O_5 and O_6 from children at Language Levels 2 and 3 in the Social Work/Supportive Counselling Group B is rejected. There was no significant difference in their performance (see above p. 110).
   Hypothesis VIIIc That children at Language Level 1 in the Speech Therapy Group C perform differently on the Reynell Expressive Language Age Test at observation points O_3, O_4, O_5 and O_6 from children at Language Levels 2 and 3 in the Speech Therapy Group C is rejected. There was no significant difference in their performance (see above p. 113).
   Hypothesis VIIId That children at Language Level 1 in the Language Programme only Group D perform differently on the Reynell Expressive Language Age Test at observation points O_3, O_4, O_5 and O_6 from children at Language Levels 2 and 3 in the Language Programme only Group D is rejected. There was no significant difference in their performance (see above p. 113).

THE RELIABILITY AND STABILITY OF IQ SCORES

Preliminary Considerations
(i) **Standardised IQ Tests and "threshold levels"**
   The study of the intellectually handicapped indicates that there is a certain "IQ threshold value" that varies with age. It is considered to be a level that must be attained for these children to acquire language (Gould 1976). However, it is noteworthy that this threshold is relatively low and that the majority of children in this study were at or above the so-called "threshold level".
   There is much research which suggests that formal tests of intelligence for the intellectually handicapped are not universally good predictors of their future *social* efficiency (Bayley 1970). Fromm and Hartman (1955) have stressed that intelligence is the dynamic functioning part of personality, and is "related to feelings, attitudes, moods, life experiences, illness, and leads no life of its own". Certainly these affective factors at the time of testing could account for variance in IQ scores of children in this sample. This point of view has been

119

supported by Spitz (1963), Decarie (1965), Inhelder (1968) and Blount (1971). They question the relevance of IQ scores for the intellectually handicapped and indicate that there are probably better ways of measuring children's capacity for intelligent behaviour; for example, measures of the maturation of the nervous system and endocrine systems (Piaget and Inhelder 1969), particularly as they relate to the co-ordination of vision and skill in the actions performed upon objects, or measures of social interaction and ability to adapt to "external disturbances" or varying exterior stimuli. However, these other methods are involved and non-standardised. As such, the children in this study have been tested on the revised Stanford Binet (Form LM) at the commencement and termination of the programmes and these IQ scores have been correlated and a distribution of IQ score changes has been prepared because:

(a) the nature of the initial discussions with parents (see Chapter 1 and Chapter 3) concerning both effective and *acceptable* means of measuring their children's performance, indicated a preference for a "traditional measure". Both Stott (1972) and Johnson (1979) indicate that whatever criticisms there are of IQ measures, they are still regarded by parents as an acceptable (if not *the* acceptable) means of assessing performance;
(b) Clarke and Clarke (1974) point out how IQ scores despite their limitations, are still the most commonly used means of classifying the moderate and severely retarded;
(c) correlation coefficients between IQ scores at different times would be a guide to the reliability of the pre-test IQ scores;
(d) it was helpful in research of this nature to guarantee that the subject population was comparable with populations in similar research (Abramowicz and Richardson 1975).
(e) individual and group mean IQ scores on a pre-test — post-test basis **may** provide some guide as to the quality of children's performances in the language areas in different treatment groups, or indeed be a guide in the qualitative evaluation of the effectiveness of different treatment programmes.

(ii) Correlation coefficients as indicators of consistency of performance

Clarke and Clarke (1975) have pointed out how important it is to be careful about the interpretation of the significance of correlation coefficients. For example, high correlations ($r = +0.9$) can give a false sense of security concerning the consistency of IQ measurements. In fact, even very high re-test correlations may conceal minorities who show large changes. Some writers, such as Bloom (1964), regard a correlation of 0.50 or above, over a period of development, as indicating the existence of a stable characteristic. However, this value implies that each measure, for example Stanford Binet IQ scores at observation points O_1 and O_6 account for only a quarter of the other's variance. Therefore, even correlations of 0.50 could imply a considerable change of status by many children in a group. Thus a correlation of 0.50 between IQ scores at different times, describes a situation with respect to these scores, which, should be regarded as much variable as consistent. Nevertheless, McCall *et al.* (1972) provide evidence that IQ correlations over time for the mentally retarded are high. Yet they also treat even these high correlations with caution, not least because high IQ correlations ($r = +0.8$) for clinical samples of the mentally retarded may merely reflect the presence of some subjects whose deficiencies are so marked that there is practically no behaviour to assess at either age.

Results: Correlation Coefficients Between Pre-test and Post-test IQ Scores

Pearson product movement correlation coefficients (Glass and Stanley, 1970) were computed for the pre-test and post-test Stanford Binet (Form LM) IQ scores (see Table 5.22). A table illustrating the distribution of changes in IQ scores has been prepared (see below Table 5.24 and p. 123).

The correlation between Stanford Binet IQ tests given at observation points O_1 and O_6 (see Table 5.23) suggested the following:
(i) that the correlation for the total sample (N=66) of $r = +0.63$ and the correlation for all girls (N=27) of $r = +0.58$ indicated a moderate relationship between IQ scores at observation

TABLE 5.22

Stanford Binet IQ Scores at Observation Points O_1 and O_6;
Table of Means and Standard Deviations.*

Group	N	O_1 CA in months M	S.D.	O_1 IQ M	S.D.	O_6 CA in months M	O_6 IQ M	S.D.
All Boys	39	86	26	38.6	8.6	119	39.8	8.9
All Girls	27	70	31	41.7	10.2	103	41.2	5.1
All Down's Syndrome	41	74	30	40.1	9.7	107	39.1	5.6
Brain Damaged	8	94	30	37.4	5.9	127	40.3	6.6
+ Mentally Handicapped	10	98	23	42.5	11.3	131	43.4	10.7
o Under 5's	23	49	7	40.4	9.8	82	40.4	7.5
Over 5's	43	100	22	39.6	8.8	133	40.4	7.6
Total Sample	66	79	30	39.9	9.4	112	40.4	7.6

* The children with IQ scores at O_1 and O_6 were considered to be representative of the total sample. The children excluded were either too young at O_1 (less than 2½ years of age) or were not available for testing at O_1. The children included here were also those children who were still in the programme at O_6.

+ There was no evidence of organic damage for this group of children. They were therefore classified as mentally handicapped of "no known organic origin".

o Children over 2½ years of age but under 5 years of age at observation point O_1.

TABLE 5.23

Correlation Coefficients Between I Q Scores at Observation Points O_1 and O_6

Group	N	O_1 CA in months M	O_1 IQ M	O_1 IQ S.D.	O_6 IQ M	O_6 IQ S.D.	Correlation Coefficient r
All Boys	39	86	38.6	8.2	39.8	8.8	0.71 ++
All Girls	27	70	41.7	10.2	41.2	5.1	0.58 ++
All Down's Syndrome	41	74	40.1	9.4	39.1	5.6	0.75 ++
Brain Damaged	8	94	37.4	5.9	40.3	6.6	0.33
ø Mentally Handicapped	10	98	42.5	11.3	43.4	10.7	0.95 ++
o Under 5's	23	49	40.4	9.8	40.4	7.5	0.33
Over 5's	43	100	39.6	8.8	40.4	7.6	0.81 ++
Total Sample	66	79	39.9	9.2	40.4	7.6	0.63 ++

ø There was no evidence of organic damage for this group of children. They were therefore classified as mentally handicapped of "no known organic origin".

o Children over 2½ years of age but under 5 years of age at observation point O_1.

++ $p < .01$ one tailed

points 0_1 and 0_6. The correlation coefficients were not sufficiently high, so that the possibility of marked changes, (e.g. a gain score of 31 IQ points or a loss of 24 IQ points (see Appendix VI)), in the IQ scores of individual children during this 33 month period, or over a longer period was precluded;

(ii) that the correlation for all boys (N=39) of $r = +0.71$, all Down's syndrome children (N=39) of $r = +0.75$, and all children over five years chronological age at the start of the programme (N=43) of $r = +0.81$, were quite high. There was therefore, an indication of stability and constancy in their IQ scores over this time period. Indeed, comparison of the correlation coefficients during this 33 months period between children **under** five years of age (N=23, mean CA 4 years 1 month, $r = +0.33$) and children **over** five years of age (N=43, mean CA 8 years 4 months, $r = +0.81$) showed clearly the increase in IQ test score constancy with increasing age. This finding is in line with Bayley's summarisation that test scores of mental growth taken in the first few years of life have relatively little reliability in contrast to tests given at school age or later (Bayley 1970);

(iii) that children whose intellectual handicap had no known organic origin (N=10) had a particularly high correlation coefficient ($r = 0.95$). As such they represented a comparatively stable group. They were however, an older group (mean CA at observation point 0_1 of 8 years 2 months, see above Table 5.22) and therefore, it was again possible to note a marked increase in their IQ correlation coefficient with increasing age. This result also indicated that the results of the IQ test given at observation point 0_1 to this particular sample were most reliable;

(iv) that children who were classified as brain damaged (N=8) had a relatively low correlation coefficient ($r = +0.33$) as had the sample of intellectually handicapped children under five years CA at the start of the programme ($r = +0.33$). As indicated above, the earlier IQ tests are given, the more likely are they to be poor predictors of the child's later performance. It also appeared that there was little reliability in IQ performance for children classified as brain damaged. Even with this small sample (N=8) there was quite a marked fluctuation in performance between tests (e.g. a gain of 17 IQ points compared with a loss of 9 IQ points (see Appendix VI)).

Distribution of IQ Score Changes

In their longitudinal study examining the stability of mental test performance between two and eighteen years, Honzik, Macfarlane and Allen (1971) write about changes in Stanford Binet IQ scores of as much as 20 points that can occur, for example, between the tests given at six and seven years. They go on to suggest that it would be reasonable to expect rather marked changes in scores over the entire test period of 18 years. Since parents are frequently concerned about likely changes in measured IQ scores (Stott 1972; Johnson 1979), a distribution of IQ score changes for the period of testing has been prepared (see Table 5.24).

An analysis of IQ changes over this 33 month period illustrated the following:

(i) that the majority of children in the all boys group, the mentally handicapped group, and children **over** five years CA group showed little change (four or less IQ points). Furthermore, the majority of the total sample (62 per cent) changed their IQ scores by four or less IQ points with only 10.6 per cent achieving changes of ten or more IQ points. This result tended to confirm the findings of Hindley and Owen (1978) who showed that at least 50 per cent of their random sample of subjects from varied social backgrounds changed their IQ scores by less than ten points over a period of nine years between test and re-test;

(ii) that the girls show a greater propensity for change in IQ scores than the boys. This may be due to their lower chronological age. However, this contrasts with earlier findings in a study of a random sample of a population by McCall et al. (1972) in which there appeared to be greater predictability in IQ scores for girls than for boys;

(iii) that the younger group (below five years of age) showed a greater propensity for change than the older group (above five years of age);

(iv) that the brain damaged group showed least stability, least constancy. Yet this was a very small sample (N=8) and while it did confirm previous findings (Knoblock and Pasamanick

TABLE 5.24

Distribution of Stanford Binet IQ Score Changes Between Observation Point O_1 and Observation Point O_6 for Different Groupings of Intellectually Handicapped Children.

Stanford Binet IQ changes between observation points O_1 and O_6	All Boys	All Girls	Down's Syndrome	Brain Damaged	Mentally Handicapped ∅	Under 5 yrs	Over 5 yrs	Total Sample
	n=39 %	n=27 %	n=41 %	n=8 %	n=10 %	n=23 %	n=43 %	n=66 %
30 or more IQ points	2.5	-	-	-	-	4.3	-	1.5
25 or more IQ points	-	-	-	-	-	-	-	-
20 or more IQ points	-	3.7	2.4	-	-	8.7	-	3.0
15 or more IQ points	-	7.4	-	12.5	-	-	2.3	4.5
10 or more IQ points	5.0	18.5	15.0	-	-	26.0	7.0	10.6
5 or more IQ points	28.0	52.0	49.0	62.5	20.0	48.0	33.0	38.0
4 or less IQ points	72.0	48.0	51.0	37.5	80.0	52.0	67.0	62.0

∅ There was no evidence of organic damage for this group of children. They were therefore classified as mentally handicapped of "no known organic origin".

1967) it was important to stress that the scores of many brain damaged children changed only slightly between pre and post-tests;

(v) that there was evidence (see Table 5.24 and Appendix VI) of marked changes in IQ scores (15 or more points) in 4.5 per cent of the total sample. For example, gain scores of 17 and 31 points, or, a loss of 24 points were reported (see Appendix VI). This is in line with the careful studies of Sontag, Baker and Nelson (1958). They have underlined the highly idiosyncratic nature of individual growth curves. As such, some individuals have periods of loss in IQ followed by a period of relatively little change. However, it is equally important to emphasise that the IQ scores of over 60 per cent of intellectually handicapped children in this sample changed only slightly (changes of 4 or less IQ points) from one age period to the next, or that over 85 per cent changed their IQ scores by less than ten IQ points.

Discussion of Results of IQ Score Correlations

The formal testing at different times to obtain a particular IQ score has resulted in some clear indication of general stability of the children's IQ scores. However, as certain individual cases indicate, this IQ score was not fixed, immutable or unchanging. Evidence existed that even for those children classified as "severely retarded", their IQ score, changed over time, and, changed with growth and experience and possibly with specific interventions. As such, for these children's parents the IQ score may be regarded as a measure of a child's current repertoire of acquired skills and knowledge. This understanding was important because even the slightest change in IQ score (particularly an improvement) was taken as an indication of a child's improved ability to acquire self-care skills, possibly to better understand language and also to talk and express himself or herself. This indication of improvement in ability in turn affected parents' motivation in caring for and teaching their children. As such, educational intervention was then considered by parents to be more effective. This then resulted in noticeable improvements in certain children's ability to learn and to progress both socially and educationally. This is a circular argument, but a most relevant one.

While it is likely that both the concept of intelligence and its measurement through standardised tests will continue to function as a critical factor in the understanding of intellectual handicap, its use is also likely to continue to affect parents' motivation to become involved in teaching their children skills.

THE RELATIONSHIP BETWEEN MEASURES OF INTELLIGENCE AND LANGUAGE DEVELOPMENT

Preliminary Considerations

Conflicting Hypotheses.

Much controversy concerns the relationship between intelligence and the acquisition of language. A recurrent question is whether a child's level of intelligence determines his or her ability to acquire language. The controversy is complicated by definitions of the nature of intelligence and is compounded by changes in intelligence quotients for the intellectually handicapped that occur with increasing chronological age (Melyn and White 1973). In addition, studies of the language behaviour of intellectually handicapped children have led to two conflicting hypotheses: (i) that these children develop language in the same sequence as normally developing children but at a much slower rate; (ii) that the sequence of development differs from that of normal children because of differences in language-processing strategies. Theoretically, of course, language delay *per se* may also result in language deviance.

In general, many conflicting statements about the language development of intellectually handicapped children appear in the literature (see above Ch. 2). Statements are made by those experimenters who claim that language development takes place in a normal sequence but at a much slower rate, and that when no further development is observed the intellectually handicapped child *has* less than the normally developing child *has* at a very much younger age. How much the retarded child *has* depends on his degree of intellectual handicap, as indicated by his measured intelligence (Lenneberg 1966). Piaget in his theory of intelligence (Piaget 1963; Piaget 1971; Piaget and Inhelder 1971), has long maintained the primacy of action or logic or, more precisely of logical mathematical structures over perceptual and symbolic structures (which include language). However, it is not clear that measured intelligence accurately predicted the linguistic performance of these children. Studies in which the correlation between linguistic performance of intellectually handicapped children and their performance on intelligence tests was examined showed that, depending on the aspect of language measured, there was a either a high or low correlation (Yoder and Miller 1972). For example, in Yoder and Miller's study, the correlation between vocabulary and IQ was +0.72, but the correlation between type/token ratio in spontaneous speech and IQ was +0.04. Similar discrepancies exist even when, presumably, the same aspect of linguistic performance is being measured. The correlations between mean length of sentence and IQ have been found to be +0.17, +0.42, and +0.68 in different studies (Yoder and Miller 1972).

A study of the development of the first 50 one-word utterances of 18 normal children by Nelson (1973) showed strong correlations between tests of intelligence and measures of language acquisition up to age 24 months. However, the correlations were considered to be "weak" at 30 months. One might infer; (i) that only at a very early stage are language and measured intelligence strongly related, or (ii) that the assessment measures of language and intelligence used were inadequate, or (iii) that the relation between measures of language and intelligence was only evident at the extremes and therefore no linear correlation existed.

Correlations between IQ scores and measured language performance

These conflicting findings may be because of the nature of the question each study asked, so that different correlations would occur, depending on whether measured IQ scores were correlated with use of spontaneous language, with specific criterion referenced language tasks, or with standardised tests used to evaluate language. Furthermore, conflicting findings may occur if the fact that intellectually handicapped children differ from each other as much as they differ from normally developing children is not taken into account, or indeed, that it is most difficult to obtain reliable test results up to a chronological age of 30 months.

The aim of this part of the study was to examine the relationship between measured intelligence and measured receptive and expressive language performance on a standardised test.

RESULTS

Pearson product moment correlation coefficients (Glass and Stanley 1970, Ch.7) were computed for different groups of intellectually handicapped children to examine the relationship between:

- Stanford Binet IQ scores and Reynell Receptive Language Age (RRLA) scores at observation point O_1.
- Stanford Binet IQ scores and Reynell Expressive Language Age (RELA) scores at observation point O_1.
- Stanford Binet IQ scores at observation point O_1 and Reynell Receptive Language Age (RRLA) scores at observation point O_6.
- Stanford Binet IQ scores at observation point O_1 and Reynell Expressive Language Age (RELA) scores at observation point O_6.
- Stanford Binet IQ scores and Reynell Receptive Language Age (RRLA) scores at observation point O_6.
- Stanford Binet IQ scores and Reynell Expressive Language Age (RELA) scores at observation point O_6.

In addition, the mean RRLA and RELA language delay for the total sample and each sub-group was calculated. This language delay is the difference between the mean RRLA or RELA scores in months and the mean CA in months at either observation point O_1 or observation point O_6 (see Table 5.28).

The results indicated:

(i) that overall there was a statistically significant relationship between measured IQ scores and measures of children's receptive and expressive language (Table 5.27). The significant correlation coefficients ($p<0.05$ to $p<0.01$) at observation point O_1 range from $r = +0.80$ (IQ score and RRLA score for mentally handicapped children) to $r = +0.37$ (IQ score and RELA score for all Down's Syndrome children) or at observation point O_6 from $r = +0.73$ (IQ score and RRLA score for mentally handicapped and brain damaged children) to $r = +0.42$ (IQ score and RELA score for the total sample). On this basis there was a clear indication that measured IQ score may be regarded as an indicator of language performance;

(ii) that IQ scores at the commencement of the programme correlate positively and significantly with RRLA and RELA scores at *both* the commencement and termination of the programme (see Table 5.27). For example, the significant correlation coefficients between measured IQ score at observation point O_1 and receptive and expressive language age at observation point O_6 range from $r = +0.71$ (for the over 5's RRLA) to $r = +0.48$ (for the under 5's age group RRLA score). On this basis, over this limited 33 month period the measured IQ score at observation point O_1 may be regarded as a useful *predictor* of children's future receptive and expressive language performance;

(iii) that the pattern of IQ scores as predictors of language age was most strong for the mentally handicapped group (of no known organic origin) and the over 5's age group. As indicated in Tables 5.25 and 5.26, these groups were also the oldest. It is reasoned therefore that the older the group, the closer was the IQ score to being a predictor of language performance. For example, the correlation coefficients for Down's Syndrome children's RRLA score and measured IQ score increased from $r = +0.39$ at observation point O_1 to $r = +0.52$ at observation point O_6;

(iv) that the correlation coefficients between measured IQ scores and RRLA scores were (with one exception out of 24 correlation coefficients) *always* higher than the correlation coefficients between measured IQ scores and RELA scores. Some subgroups in particular illustrated contrasting correlation coefficients between measured IQ and RRLA and/or RELA scores. For example, at observation point O_1 the correlation coefficient for IQ and RRLA for mentally handicapped children $r = +0.80$ whereas for IQ and RELA $r = +0.35$. Similarly at observation point O_6 the correlation coefficients for IQ and RRLA for all girls $= +0.51$ whereas for IQ and RELA $r = +0.29$. It may be reasoned therefore that an IQ score was a better predictor of children's measured receptive language performance than it was of their measured expressive language performance;

(v) that as all these intellectually handicapped children get older so their *language delay* increased (see Table 5.28). This receptive and expressive language delay was smallest for the younger groups, (the under 5's, all Down's Syndrome children), and greatest for the older groups, (the familial mentally handicapped (of no known organic origin) and the over 5's, (see Table 5.28)). The average RRLA score lag at observation point O_1 for children with a mean CA of 6 years 7 months was 3 years 9 months, and the RELA score lag was 4 years 7 months. Thirty-three months later when the mean CA was 9 years 4 months, the RRLA score lag had increased to 5 years 9 months and the RELA score lag to 6 years 2 months.

(vi) Only the small group of brain damaged subjects ($N=8$) failed to show a statistically significant difference between the measured RRLA and RELA delay scores at observation points O_1 and O_6 (see Table 5.28). Thirteen of the fourteen other receptive and expressive language delay scores demonstrated a significant difference ($p<0.05$) between measured receptive and expressive language delays at observation point O_1 when compared with measured receptive and expressive language delays at observation point O_6.

Discussion of Results: The relationship between IQ measures and language development.

The correlation coefficients indicated that for this sample of intellectually handicapped children there was a close relationship between IQ score and language development. However, there was a definite indication that receptive language development was much more closely tied to IQ scores than expressive language development. In particular, for the small group of brain damaged children, expressive language development appeared to be even more independent of IQ scores than for any other group of intellectually handicapped children.

TABLE 5.25

Reynell Developmental Language Age Observed Scores in Months for Receptive and Expressive Language at Observation Point O_1

Table of Means and Standard Deviations

Group	N	CA		RRLA		RELA	
		M mths	S.D. mths	M mths	S.D. mths	M mths	S.D. mths
All Boys	39	86	26	35	13.8	25	13.2
All Girls	27	70	31	33	15.3	24	13.6
All Down's Syndrome	41	74	30	32	13.7	24	12.8
Brain Damaged	8	94	23	37	14.2	29	13.8
+ Mentally Handicapped	10	98	23	41	14.3	29	14.6
o Under 5's	23	49	7	24	9.8	17	8.1
Over 5's	43	100	22	39	13.8	29	13.8
Total Sample	66	79	30	34	14.5	25	13.4

+ There was no evidence of organic damage for this group of children. They were therefore classified as mentally handicapped of "no known organic origin".

o Children over 2½ years of age but under 5 years of age at observation point O_1.

TABLE 5.26

Reynell Developmental Language Age Observed Scores in Months for Receptive and Expressive Language at Observation Point O_6

Table of Means and Standard Deviations

Group	N	CA		RRLA		RELA	
		M mths	S.D. mths	M mths	S.D. mths	M mths	S.D. mths
All Boys	39	119	26	43	14.4	39	15.7
All Girls	27	103	31	44	13.4	38	12.3
All Down's Syndrome	41	107	30	43	13.9	37	14.7
Brain Damaged	8	127	30	46	13.0	45	11.0
+ Mentally Handicapped	10	131	23	45	17.6	38	15.1
ø Under 5's	23	82	7	38	9.8	33	8.6
Over 5's	43	133	22	46	15.1	41	16.0
Total Sample	66	112	30	43	14.1	39	14.4

+ There was no evidence of organic damage for this group of children. They were therefore classified as mentally handicapped of "no known organic origin".

ø Children over 2½ years of age but under 5 years of age at observation point O_1.

129

TABLE 5.27

Pearson Product Moment Correlation Coefficients between Stanford Binet IQ Observed Scores and Reynell Receptive and Expressive Language Age Observed Scores at Observation Points O_1 and O_6

Group	N	Correlation Coefficient IQ at O_1 and RRLA at O_1	Correlation Coefficient IQ at O_1 and RELA at O_1	Correlation Coefficient IQ at O_1 and RRLA at O_6	Correlation Coefficient IQ at O_1 and RELA at O_6	Correlation Coefficient IQ at O_6 and RRLA at O_6	Correlation Coefficient IQ at O_6 and RELA at O_6
All Boys	39	0.49 ++	0.47 ++	0.65 ++	0.58 ++	0.52 ++	0.47 ++
All Girls	27	0.47 ++	0.31	0.52 ++	0.48 ++	0.51 ++	0.29
All Down's Syndrome	41	0.39 +	0.37 +	0.58 ++	0.51 ++	0.52 ++	0.44 ++
Brain Damaged	8	0.27	0.42	0.24	0.65	0.73 +	0.39
Mentally Handicapped	10	0.80 ++	0.35	0.77 ++	0.58	0.73 +	0.56
Under 5's	23	0.49 +	0.43 +	0.48 +	0.36 +	0.28	0.19
Over 5's	43	0.60 ++	0.47 ++	0.71 ++	0.64 ++	0.63 ++	0.52 ++
Total Sample	66	0.46 ++	0.38 ++	0.59 ++	0.51 ++	0.51 ++	0.42 ++

RRLA   Reynell Receptive Language Age   + $p < .05$ one tailed.

RELA   Reynell Expressive Language Age   ++ $p < .01$ one tailed.

TABLE 5.28

Table to Illustrate Delay* in Receptive and Expressive
Language Development at the Observation point O_1 and Observation point O_6

Group	N	Obs Time	Receptive Language Delay mths	Increase in delay at O_6 mths	Expressive Language Delay mths	Increase in delay at O_6 mths
Boys	39	O_1	51		61	
		O_6	76	25 ++	80	19 ++
Girls	27	O_1	37		46	
		O_6	59	22 ++	64	18 ++
Down's Syndrome	41	O_1	42		50	
		O_6	64	22 ++	70	20 ++
Brain Damaged	8	O_1	56		64	
		O_6	80	24	81	17
Mentally Handi-capped.		O_1	57		69	
		O_6	86	29 ++	93	24 +
Under 5s	23	O_1	24		31	
		O_6	44	20 ++	48	17 ++
Over 5's	43	O_1	57		67	
		O_6	83	26 ++	88	21 ++
Total Sample	66	O_1	45		55	
		O_6	69	24 ++	74	19 ++

* Measure of delay in language development is indicated by the difference
between CA and the mean RRLA and RELA scores at observation points O_1 and O_6.

+ $p < 0.05$ one tailed.) The t test values were calculated for the difference
++ $p < 0.01$ one tailed.) between RRLA scores and CA, and RELA scores and CA.

As with other studies it was confirmed that both delay and disturbance of language are central features of moderate to severe intellectual handicap. It was established in this testing programme that the children's language problem was not only that when their speech developed it was quite delayed, but also that for some, it was deviant (see above p. 125 and below Chapter 7). That is, characteristics such as echolalia were prominent, particularly at the one word stage, articulation difficulties abounded and defects in the understanding of spoken language, particularly at the two word stage and beyond, were widespread.

The increasing delay in both receptive and expressive language, confirmed findings in other studies. Menyuk (1976) described the sequence of stages of normal child language acquisition from the "First Stage: Before Babbling" to the "Fifth Stage: Acquisition of the Grammar of the Language". Cromer (1974) described the increasingly sophisticated and "mature" rules required for children to advance to the later stages of language acquisition. It appeared therefore that the intellectually handicapped have much difficulty in shifting from the use of primitive rules to mature rules (also see above p. 102). Since language development is clearly dependent on physiological development as well as cognitive and social development, these intellectually handicapped children had increasing difficulty in maintaining their rate of language acquisition when compared to normal subjects. Therefore, the higher order language stages in Reynell's Developmental Language Scales, particularly those requiring strategies for the "creative use of language", may be either beyond these intellectually handicapped children or they may be using different processing strategies which this particular developmental language test did not tap. Only when the language development of the intellectually handicapped is studied with the intensity and care with which normal development is being studied can the intellectually handicapped child's "language delay", or the nature and function of the intellectually handicapped child's language acquisition strategies, be more clearly defined.

In short, what has to be explained to parents of the intellectually handicapped was not only the children's limited use and understanding of language, but also the nature of the cognitive deficit which itself hindered language development. The cognitive deficit was apparent in both reduced sensorimotor alertness and ability to manipulate symbols. It also took the form of these children having difficulty in representing what was perceived, particularly when the language that was used was independent of the context in which it was used and when there was little use of gesture (see also Ch. 7).

Intellectual handicap for these children involved delay and some disorders of language which clearly involved problems of sequencing and abstraction. The correlation between intelligence and language acquisition was stronger for older children. As such, chronological age appeared to be a guide for these children's current status in language development. However, it must be emphasised that this study was concerned with examining the relationship between IQ scores and standardised language age scores. Different findings could well result if IQ scores were correlated with other measures of language acquisition, such as the use of spontaneous language, mean length of utterances, sentence or speech repetition abilities, or specific contextual language tasks.

Chapter Six

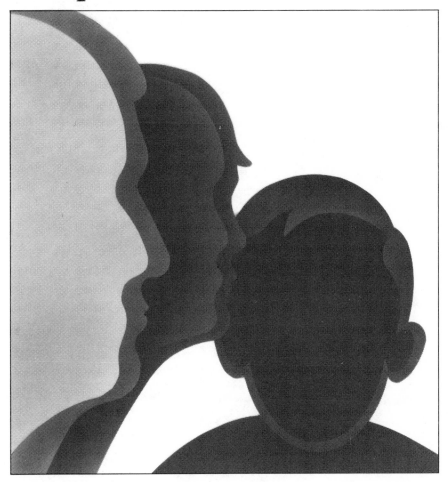

Parent Attitudes

Preliminary Considerations

It was insisted throughout this project that the successful teaching of the moderate and severely handicapped children depended on the full involvement of their parents. Indeed, parental involvement was an integral part of the project. However, because of the severe nature of their children's handicap so many of these parents had burdens to bear, of which others may have no conception. It was therefore an essential part of this programme that not only were parents advised, shown, helped and consulted, but also that their attitudes towards teaching their children were carefully surveyed. It was reasoned that an understanding and appreciation of these attitudes could make the programme more effective (see above Ch. 1 and Ch. 3). The evidence that was received in the Capital Territory Health Commission Survey of Parent Attitudes towards this language teaching programme (Kimber and Porritt, 1976, and Rees, 1978) strongly confirms this point of view. For example, a group of parents involved in the programme from the outset stated that:

We always care for our children for a longer part of the day than any professional. It is we who must endure the disruption of family and social life which an intellectually handicapped child brings. Our attitudes to the child are the key to the success of any treatment programme, and the greater the understanding by the professionals, the greater is the chance of successful co-operation. Parents will always listen to someone who is on their side in their efforts to care for and teach the child.

Just as the special language needs of the children in this programme took a great variety of forms, so did the needs of their parents. Any discussion of these needs in general terms must not be allowed to obscure the truth that they are individually "special". Despite the attempts to define common attitudes and needs and plan accordingly, no two cases were the same. The needs and attitudes of an individual parent reflected the nature of her child's handicap, particularly its degree of severity and the weight of dependence upon parental and family support that it entails. They also reflected the family circumstances. Cramped or isolated accommodation obviously severely hampered parents in looking after a young handicapped child: likewise a large family, particularly where there were young children, imposed its own constraints. Parents were more able to cope if they themselves were in good health, if there were two of them, if they were free from financial or other anxieties, and if they had helpful neighbours, relatives or friends. Equally, parents differed widely in their attitudes, temperament, insight, knowledge, teaching ability, and ability to sustain their teaching. All these factors powerfully influenced the extent and nature of the help that parents required.

It was clear that some parents merely wished from time to time to discuss their difficulties with someone else. Others required elaborate advice and help, mostly on a regular and continuing basis. Between these extremes there was a gradation of intensity and complexity of individual parental needs which were moreover dynamic and which changed with time. At the outset the programme endeavoured to provide a pattern of flexible service for parents which could be carefully evaluated and which matched the different forms of help that parents required. Special arrangements therefore had to be made to understand parent attitudes towards teaching the intellectually handicapped child at home and to enabling both parents and professionals to improve their understanding of the children's needs.

It was clear from the beginning that the expectations of parents had to be as appropriate as possible (see above, Ch. 1). During the establishment of the programme, Stage I (see above Ch. 3, p. 56), parents and professionals together decided that traditional norms were inappropriate expectations for these children. It was reasoned that if the revised goals and aspirations were drawn from the parents then they were more likely to develop the self-confidence and teaching skills necessary to maximise their child's development. Parents provided this information by: (a) their responses in open interviews (see above Ch. 3, p. 55); (b) their responses to the Parent Opinion Survey (Kimber and Porritt 1976); and (c) their completion of the Parent As A Teacher Inventory (PAAT) (Strom 1976; Strom and Slaughter 1978).

Many parents hoped for integration of their children into "normal" life situations. The success story of Roger and Virginia Myers, both retarded since birth, who married and have achieved a "normal" life, indicates the importance of parents' high expectations for their intellectually handicapped children (Myers 1978). The literature is replete with examples of successful integration (Ansol Occasional Papers No. 2 1976). However, expectations that are unrealistically high for intellectually handicapped children may lead in most cases to greater parental frustration and defeat. At the same time "commonsense", "normal" attitudes towards everyday child behaviour reflecting traditional normative value systems may also produce frustration in child handling and reduce opportunities for child learning.

The PAAT provided all parents with the opportunity of indicating and discussing these attitudes. Furthermore, attitudes highly specific to parent teaching could be attended to by the professionals working with the parents (see above Ch. 4, p. 69).

Results and Discussion

(i) Use of the PAAT total scores

The use of the PAAT total scores as an indication of parents' attitudes to working with their children requires careful examination. It appears that the PAAT total scores were a useful guide to establishing which families were likely to be "more open, innovative and persistent" and those who might be classified as "defensive, uncertain and less persistent".

Those parents with total PAAT scores at 0_2 above 150 (see Table 6.1) were most likely to be "innovative and persistent" and parents whose total PAAT score was 140 or above could also be considered to possess the same traits. In contrast, those parents whose total PAAT score was below 130, and certainly those 10 parents with scores below 120 (see Table 6.1) *tended* to be "defensive, uncertain and less persistent" in their behaviour towards their children (see also Ch. 2, p. 43).

TABLE 6.1

Distribution of Parents' Total P.A.A.T. Scores
among etiology groups

Group	Below 120 N	120-130 N	140-150 N	Above 150 N
Down's Syndrome	2	5	20	13
Brain Damaged	4	3	2	4
Epileptic	1	-	2	2
Hydrocephalic	-	-	1	-
Microcephalic	1	2	1	2
Genetic Disorder	-	1	1	1
Mentally Handicapped	2	2	2	1
Total	10	13	29	23

It needs to be emphasised that using PAAT total scores as the basis for "unidimensional" descriptions of parent attitudes is somewhat simplistic. Rather the PAAT score results and discussion with parents about their attitudes to teaching their children support Kerlinger's contention that "social attitudes of which educational attitudes are a part, are dualistic" (Kerlinger 1967) and that, according to the position a parent takes, one or two different sets of

136

issues and problems give rise to the criterion by which the parent judges his action or attitudes towards action. To use Kerlinger's own terminology, different "referents" can be "criterial" for different individuals. Therefore, parents who, with total scores above one hundred and fifty, have been described as "open, innovative and persistent" were clearly sensitive to different issues and problems or to different aspects of these problems when compared with parents with total PAAT scores below one hundred and twenty who have been described as "defensive, uncertain and less persistent".

An alternative hypothesis is that parent attitudes are fundamentally unidimensional and bipolar. As such, the basic principle in consensus building between parent and parent educators depends on the discovery of an appropriate point of a continuum which connects attitudes pleasing to parents who are "open, innovative and persistent" with one pleasing to parents who are "defensive, uncertain and less persistent". However, just as the results reported here cast doubt on the validity of assuming a good ("open, innovative and persistent") or bad ("defensive, uncertain and less persistent") dimension, so they also seem to indicate that parent attitudes towards teaching their children are just not bipolar either.

(ii) Total and Subset Means

The total and subset means for the entire sample of one hundred and one parents are shown in Table 6.2. The highest subset mean score was in the Teaching-Learning and Play subsets, with the lowest means found in the Creativity and Control subsets. The parents' total mean of 139.1 was somewhat higher than the absolute median of 125. This was within the range of means from 133.9 to 144.8 reported for various ethnic groups of parents of normal children in the United States (Strom and Slaughter, 1978). The internal reliability of the PAAT was relatively high, as indicated by an alpha coefficient of 0.85.

TABLE 6.2

P A A T Subset Means, S.D. and Internal Reliability
Coefficients for 101 Parents of Intellectually
Handicapped Children.

Subset	M	S.D.	Alpha
Creativity	26.4	3.3	.47
Frustration	27.7	3.1	.51
Control	26.3	3.2	.45
Play	29.1	3.6	.62
Teaching-Learning	29.6	4.3	.71
Total	139.1	13.5	.85

(iii) Comparison of Down's syndrome and Brain Damaged Subgroups' Total and Subset Means.

The results for the two largest subgroups, parents of children with Down's Syndrome and parents of brain damaged children, as seen in Table 6.3, indicated more positive attitudes on the part of parents of children with Down's Syndrome than of those with brain damaged children. The difference of 8.4 points between the total means was not significant (using Cochran and Cox's (1957) formula for testing the significance of the computed t when variances differ, as shown by an F test). It should be noted that the sample of Down's Syndrome children was about a

137

year younger than the brain damaged sample (Table 1.4) and this age difference could well have influenced the results. Moreover, the Down's Syndrome children had a slightly higher mean Stanford Binet IQ score (40.4) than the brain damaged children (37.4).

It is felt that chronological age is a most relevant factor. Generally parents of younger children proved to be more open and innovative, and their children's language behaviours more pliant. However, the PAAT was developed for a younger population and may be more appropriate for measuring parental attitudes about interacting with the younger child. It is essential to recognise the importance of age derived differences of the intellectually handicapped. In other words, *chronological* age, as well as "mental" age, is important in the diagnosis and assessment of this group. After all, deviant language and social behaviours may be less established in younger children (Lenneberg, 1967; Renfrew, 1972). As such, they are more open to modification and their parents are more likely to experience success in home based teaching.

TABLE 6.3

P A A T Subset Means, S.D. and Internal Reliability
Coefficients for 56 Parents of Children with
Down's Syndrome and 16 Parents of Brain
Damaged Children.

Subset	Down's Syndrome			Brain Damaged		
	M	S.D.	Alpha	M	S.D.	Alpha
Creativity	27.1	3.1	.45	25.3	3.3	.51
Frustration	28.3	2.6	.30	26.9	4.4	.80
Control	26.8	2.8	.34	25.6	3.9	.65
Play	29.7	3.4	.61	27.9	4.0	.65
Teaching-Learning	30.4	3.5	.76	28.2	5.6	.83
Total	142.3	10.3	.76	133.9	18.9	.93

(iv) Analysis of Subsets

The interpretation of subset results has been extended by the parents' personal comments during administration of the PAAT at 0_2, by recorded interviews during Stage II (see above Ch. 3) which followed the administration of the PAAT and by examining videotapes of interaction with their children in the individual language training teaching sessions (see above Ch. 3, p. 57-61).

Creativity Subset. These items allowed parents to examine issues relating to (a) encouraging children to persist at tasks; (b) valuing the privacy of the child (particularly the older handicapped child) and (c) allowing the child to express uncertainty. Furthermore, attitude statements in this subset allowed parents the opportunity to discuss alternatives for solving the developmental problems of the handicapped child. The creativity subset received relatively low scores and contained three weak items, as determined by item/total correlations. These items were not directly applicable to a non-speaking, intellectually handicapped child; for example, "When my child doesn't know an answer, I ask him to guess", or "it is alright for my child to spend a lot of time playing alone".

On one item there was definite disagreement between the PAAT preferred response and parents' preference. "I seldom tell my child his work is good or bad so that my child can make up his own mind" revealed a parental preference for telling the child that his work is good or bad. The extent to which a parent allowed or could wait for a handicapped child to "make up his own

138

mind" is often uncertain. Parents pointed out that "this can be stressful for the child", or "it can lead to much time wasting". Some stated, "No matter what the handicap, a child needs to know whether what he is doing is good or bad!" This last response indicated clearly that this sample of parents preferred a behaviour modification rather than a "creative developmental" approach to child rearing values as indicated by the PAAT preferred responses. There was clear evidence why parents preferred this response. Interviews during the first stage of the language programme (see above Ch. 3, p. 55) demonstrated parents' desire for structure in teaching and emphasised the importance of the parental role in decision making. Furthermore, in the lead up to the production of the language manual (see above Ch. 3, p. 56) parents demonstrated their preference for careful task analysis and considered selection of appropriate reinforcers. Secondly, the role expectations for these parents were created by the group leaders who initially sought the establishment of the language intervention programme. At the outset every parent was faced with conflicts in deciding what socialisation goals to strive for in the children who they loved, cared for and taught. Seventy five per cent of these parents revealed in individual interviews (see Ch. 4, p. 69) that they were concerned about their handicapped children having opportunities to "be creative". However, very few of them wanted this desire for creativity to be extended to "bizarre extremes". "Parents have to be authoritative" explained a parent of a retarded six year old, hence the reaction to the statement "I seldom tell my child his work is good or bad". However, it should not be construed that these parents were authoritarian or that they regarded this particular PAAT statement as "permissive". Rather these parents formulated goals for their children clearly and also, despite the children's limitations, had great respect for the integrity and ingenuity of the children. As such, their expressed attitudes to such PAAT statements indicated what they considered to be the most effective way of achieving both language and socialisation goals for their children. This parental behaviour was identical with that of parents of normal four year olds studied by Baumrind (1971). In this study Baumrind demonstrated that the most autonomous and socially responsible of the many four year olds she studied came from homes where parents were authoritative, but not authoritarian and not permissive. Parents in this programme through their interactions with their children and responses to the PAAT demonstrated that they too were concerned to be authoritative.

Frustration Subset. The frustration subset was designed to help parents clarify their child rearing expectations and indicate those behaviours which they judged to be upsetting. It is postulated that frustration in child rearing (particularly for parents of the intellectually handicapped) can be reduced by understanding why certain child behaviours occur and the reason why some of them should be permitted.

When responding to the frustration subset, parents pointed out that caring for an intellectually handicapped child automatically means that a family providing such care was bound to be different in some ways from families who did not have an intellectually handicapped child. This difference can be seen not just in terms of the greater amount of care, but also, as many subjects pointed out, in the emotional attitude that parents and siblings have towards the intellectually handicapped child. For many families, a critical aspect was the extent to which they were emotionally bound up with the intellectually handicapped child. At one end of the scale, the intellectually handicapped child appeared to be the centre of his or her parents' lives to the exclusion of all else. The other end of the scale involved homes where the child was not the emotional centre of the family, and they were not totally bound up with him or her. Yet, at the same time, the child was loved and valued. These families generally demonstrated that they had many contacts in the community with friends and neighbours. For them the frustration subset statements were highly relevant. Their intellectually handicapped children were quite involved in everyday life, rather than hidden away in little worlds of their own.

The locus of frustration for parents of intellectually handicapped children is best expressed by the comment, "I want my child to be able to talk". As such, some frustration subset statements may appear quite peripheral to those behaviours of the intellectually handicapped child which must frustrate parents. In common with parents' responses to commenting on their children's work or behaviour in the creativity subset (see above, p. 138) parents here showed a concern for "order in the household" by the majority of their "Strong Yes" replies to the statement, "I want my child to put the toys away before going to bed". This response again contrasts with the PAAT criteria for the "most desirable response". However, for many parents, irrespective of their treatment group, the subset statements did provide a locus of frustration and, as such, they enabled parents to indicate that their attitudes would be the *same* for their handicapped children as for their nonhandicapped children.

Modifying parental expectations is something that parents of intellectually handicapped children have to accept. "You've got to accept them for what they are and not keep wishing they were normal", said a father of an eight year old Down's Syndrome boy. Time after time this point about acceptance of the child and modification of expectations was made. Certainly, in any educational programme for parents of handicapped children, the frustration subset could form a basis for discussing with parents the modification of their expectations. However, sixty per cent of parents pointed out that if a family was to cope with an intellectually handicapped child at home for the length of time that many of them had *adjustments in expectations* will take place *naturally*.

Control Subset. This subset focused on parent feelings about dominance and the extent to which their control of child behaviour was deemed necessary. The statements included two relatively weak items, and parents' mean scores were low (see Table 6.2 and Appendix VII).

It is clear that parents of intellectually handicapped children are often perplexed about the amount of control they should exercise over their children. The problem is one of balance. As one parent put it, "It is disastrous to be too accepting of B's behaviour (you give up trying to control him if you are); equally, it is disastrous to be constantly dissatisfied with him ... trying to *control* his every action ... then you don't make the best use of what you have". This was the dilemma of parental control which the PAAT posed, even though some of its statements about control ("While we play, my child should be the person in control" or "I provide chances for my child to make up his own mind about a lot of things") were clearly more applicable to parental interaction with a non-handicapped child. Nevertheless, parents' responses to these statements demonstrated that in many, many cases the fact of having an intellectually handicapped child did not alter their responses. Some parents did recognise that for these children there can be no favourable self-impression without some feeling of control, and that learning to sense power and to share dominance with parents and other members of the family are important ingredients for mental health.

Issues raised by such statements as "It's alright for my child to disagree with me" or "I like my child to be quiet when adults are talking" or "I provide chances for my child to make up his own mind about a lot of things" led to parental discussion about the relationship between adult control and the need of the intellectually handicapped child for developing some measure of independence. Independence for the adolescent handicapped child depends so much on his early preparation for this, as well as on his developing language and communication skills. Parents' responses to this subset revealed that some were concerned that too much parental control would result in the child growing up with *little* independence. Seventy-five per cent of responses revealed a definite concern for generating an atmosphere at home where, through play, through establishing consequences for actions that are non-punitive, through an atmosphere of mutual respect, the child would grow up confident, secure and, hopefully, more independent. Interviews with these parents demonstrated that they were concerned with models of normality and excellence rather than with models of abnormality and **pathology**. As such, they emphasised their children's positive growth and the importance of prosocial behaviour. The process by which this prosocial behaviour could be achieved depended on "a parent having control" and on being able to "teach prosocial skills". This heterogeneous group of parents were not in agreement about "how much control" they should exercise or exactly which prosocial skills "were most desirable" apart from the recurring theme of "being able to talk or communicate". However, they were most accepting of the importance of endeavouring to share decision making with their children as well as allowing for disagreement and privacy.

Play Subset. This subset refers to parental understanding of play and its influence on child development. When interviewed parents were clear about the kind of play their children participated in, where different objects are manipulated in the same way. For example, there are certain actions that can be performed on objects regardless of the different perceptual properties or different functions that different objects might have. Then the children learned that objects with different textures or tastes could nevertheless be mouthed or eaten, or that many objects could be dropped, thrown or banged. However, parents pointed out that their children had "great difficulty" with object-specific play (see above Ch. 2, p. 29). That is, there are certain actions that can be performed with only certain objects, depending on the perceptual properties and functions that different objects have. For example, only paper can be crumpled; a ball rolled. The intellectually handicapped child's difficulties in play appear at the stage where a distinction has to be made between object-specific play and nonspecific play. Bricker and Bricker (1974) in their early language intervention programme stressed the importance of learning the nonlinguistic behaviour that is preliminary to learning language behaviours. They reported a comparison between two groups of two year old children playing with objects, one a group of mentally retarded children, and the other, a group of children developing normally. The retarded children used more nonspecific play behaviours, while the normally developing children used more object-specific play.

The numerous studies of children's play life reported in psychological literature have provided much valuable data on this important phase of child development. However, most of these studies have been concerned with varied aspects of the play activities of normal children of preschool and primary ages (Bruner et al 1976). Bruner (1972) writes that play can be a means of minimising the consequences of one's actions and of learning, therefore, in a less risky situation; in addition, play provides an excellent opportunity to try combinations of behaviour that would, under functional pressure, never be tried.

These aspects of play are vital to the social development of intellectually handicapped children. Strom (1978) describes the importance of the pretending role in play and an account of this appears in this subset. Vygotsky (1966) and Piaget (1951) demonstrate the relationship between fantasy play in the young and its impact on creative activity at a later age. We may ask whether this is of relevance to intellectually handicapped children. Parent responses to this subset demonstrated an appreciation of all these points. However, it does appear that there is a greater need for *specificity* in the play of the intellectually handicapped; that is, a programme in which the child is *trained* in specific perceptual and social skills. This need was emphasised by Jeffree and McConkey (1976b) in their writing about the relationship between play and the development of language in the intellectually handicapped.

The responses of parents to the play subset statements emphasised a distinction between the different nature of play for a normal child and an intellectually handicapped child. For example, children who easily engage in fantasy play are more able to concentrate, persist at tasks, and are better able to cope with anxiety (Strom, 1978). Parents in the sample demonstrated an appreciation of this benefit in their response to such statements as, "My Child needs to play with me" or "My child learns by playing with other children". However, the qualitative difference in the nature of play with an intellectually handicapped child was emphasised by parents in their response to such statements as, "Playing with my child makes me feel restless" or "My child learns new words when we play", or more particularly, "It is difficult for me to stay interested when playing with my child". These items received a consistent low score in the responses. Moreover, discussion with parents, along with observation of their behaviour, demonstrated the close relationship between their expressed difficulties and the problems that they had in playing with their children.

Discussion about the play subset items revealed that parents appreciated the importance of play. Yet, in many cases, they were confused by, on the one hand, the relationship between understanding the importance of a broad programme of play activities in meeting the problems of recreation and adjustment for their intellectually handicapped child, and on the other, the child's persistnt stereotyped responses in situations where the ingenuity of a normal child may have been more reinforcing and motivating to the parent. This conflict represented real frustration for the parent; furthermore, the qualitative difference clearly affected a parent's readiness to participate in the favourite play activity of an intellectually handicapped child. Any parent

141

intervention programme needs to take this into account and endeavour to train that object-specific play, which is such a vital precursory goal, of both language form and content.

Teaching-Learning Subset. This group of items was concerned with parental perception of their ability to facilitate the teaching-learning process. Parents' scores were highest on this subset and the group contained only one weak item.

For many years, parents of intellectually handicapped children were led to believe that they did not have the necessary ability to help their children learn, and were discouraged from doing so by policies of institutionalising the child from as early an age as possible (Lustig 1977; Payne 1976; Pueschel and Murphy 1975). Later, when studies began to suggest the importance of early environment (Bronfenbrenner 1974), it did seem that the teaching possibilities of parents of the intellectually handicapped (given adequate backup services) were again overlooked. These early programmes seldom made provision for meaningful parent involvement. However, there has been a dramatic shift in emphasis so that the present situation is one which increasingly recognises the unique possibilities of parent influence. Indeed, there is even a journal in the U.S.A. called *The Exceptional Parent.*

Given the ideal of individualised instruction, it was important to recognise that the family has the most desirable teacher-pupil ratio. Then, too, parents are the primary teachers while an intellectually handicapped child lives at home. But to successfully teach verbal skills, parents need self-confidence and instructional procedures pertinent to the child's level of language development. Responses to the teaching-learning subset and mother-father comments on the items reveal the following:

1. That over 80 per cent of parents accept their child's intellectual handicap and as such did not "deny reality". However, this acceptance does not alter their responses to their views about "their child having a make believe friend" or to their use of toys when they play with their child. Parents indicated that responses to these items would be similar, if not identical, if they were responding to statements about teaching their non-handicapped child.

2. That parents were generally not over-protective toward their handicapped child. They genuinely wanted to try to teach, even though the majority of them saw themselves as unable to provide the necessary learning experiences at home. Two factors determined this point of view. One was that most parents were very aware of the importance of early education. Mindful of what they regarded as their inadequate background, parents of these children were especially apprehensive about doing a poor job. Lacking a knowledge of the behavioural norms for boys and girls of their child's condition, the parents felt uncertain about what goals and expectations were appropriate (see above Ch. 3, p. 55). For some families the ambiguity was resolved by turning all educational decisions over to the professionals who, they supposed, understood the norms. While the overreliance on professionals was intended to be in the child's best interest, it could also prevent the unique benefits which both parties gained from parent-child interaction.

    The opposite experience of some parents inhibited their participation in teaching. These families had consulted with a variety of professionals who seldom seemed to agree with one another. Believing that they had frequently been provided with misinformation, the parents expressed serious reservations about how much experts in fact really knew about handicapped children. For example, at the one extreme, some professionals have led parents to erroneously believe that the child would "outgrow" his condition. Other parents referred to comments that their child's condition was diagnosed as "near hopeless" with immediate institutionalisation as the only solution. It seems some professionals do generate self-fulfilling and self-limiting prophecies which mitigate against the parents actively teaching their intellectually handicapped child. Despite the desire to teach their children and maximise development, mothers and fathers were, and are, very sensitive to such defeatist attitudes.

3. That parents were accepting of the idea of the use of toys in teaching their children language skills. Their responses to the statement, "It is easy for me to use toys when teaching my child" demonstrated their ready acceptance of this medium. Access to toy talk methods

(Strom, 1978), toy lending libraries and the guidance of speech therapists with younger intellectually handicapped children enhanced this possibility.

4. That in the teaching situation seventy per cent of the parents indicated that they did *not* find it difficult to tell when their child had learned something.
5. That parents were quite aware of the affective reactions of the intellectually handicapped child to success and failure. This was shown by responses to such statements as, "I scold my child when he does not learn" or "If we play whenever my child wants to, not much learning will take place". Furthermore, parent responses again revealed a very great respect for their children and real *concern* to develop their own teaching skills. Discussion of these items with parents also revealed that their intellectually handicapped children were often quite sensitive to, and capable of, identifying parents' feelings towards them in the teaching-learning situation. However, parents were clear that very little had previously been offered to assist them in "techniques of child management, stimulation and teaching programmes". Indeed discussion of these Teaching-Learning subset items revealed the quite heavy financial, personal and emotional commitment of many families to controversial programmes for which great claims are made (see above Ch. 2, p. 18). This demonstrated both the extent to which families searched for means of teaching their children and the dearth of options open to them. This is important because even by the end of the specific teaching programme at 0_5 (see above Ch. 3, Fig. 3.1) seventy-four per cent of parents expressed the point of view that they were still *not* able to give their children the necessary teaching experience at home. Parents were concerned that even though they had demonstrated their ability to teach their children at home, any specific parent recognition or acceptance of this skill could lead to a reduction in support services. Parent responses to the Teaching-Learning subset revealed that they wanted to be active participators in language teaching alongside the relevant professionals.

(v) **Attitudes and behaviours of parents most and least successful in the language training programme and some characteristics of their children.**

The total PAAT score for parents scoring at either the upper or lower extremes proved to be an excellent guide for identifying individual parents who were most and least successful in the Language Training Programme. For example, twenty-three parents whose total mean score was 150 or more proved to be parents who:

1. maintained an 80 per cent or better attendance record at the parent group training sessions and individual teaching/therapy sessions;
2. maintained the most regular criterion records of their home-based teaching and their children, generally, were having the most success on the language tasks (see Table 6.4);
3. were most open to new ideas in teaching their children and, in particular, were most willing to be filmed in the home or clinic setting;
4. were most willing to persist with a language task even when they were obtaining little success in the early stages;
5. maintained contact and sought advice from the speech therapists during the third year of the programme (see Ch. 3, p. 61) and generally had developed patterns of seeking and using help;
6. indicated they gained personal benefit from face-to-face contact with other parents and staff in the programme.

Alternatively, ten parents whose total mean score on the PAAT was 120 or less, proved to be parents who:

1. kept to the minimum attendance record at both group training and individual teaching/therapy sessions;
2. had much difficulty in keeping regular criterion records of home-based teaching;
3. were considerably less open to new ideas;
4. found it most difficult to persist in a task;
5. made little or no contact of their own initiative with the speech therapists during the third year of the programme;

6. were generally *uncertain* as to whether their child would remain at home or, indeed, expressed uncertainty about the family/child relationship.

When the characteristics of the children of parents with high (>150) or low (<120) PAAT total scores were examined some similarities and distinct differences appeared (see Table 6.4). These were:—

(a) that the average number of children in the family for both groups of parents was three.

(b) that parents with high PAAT total scores (>150) had younger intellectually handicapped children than parents with low PAAT total scores (<120) though there was no significant difference in the chronological age of these different groups of children;

(c) that the children of parents with high PAAT total scores (>150) had a higher mean Stanford Binet measured IQ score (IQ 39.2 — SD 7.5) than the children of parents with low PAAT total scores (<120)(mean Stanford Binet measured IQ score of 33.0, SD 10.5). This difference was not statistically significant; +

(d) that the children of parents with higher PAAT total scores (>150) had higher mean measured receptive language age scores at the commencement of the programme (0_1) than the children of parents with lower mean PAAT total scores (<120) (see Table 6.4) and that after the first year of preparation for the language intervention programme (0_1 to 0_2) this difference in measured receptive language age had increased from 5.6 months to 7.6 months. However, this gain score difference was not statistically significant; +

(e) that the children of parents with higher PAAT total scores (>150) had higher mean measured expressive language age scores at the commencement of the programme (0_1) than the children of parents with lower mean PAAT total scores (<120) and that after the first year of preparation for the language intervention programme (0_1 to 0_2) this difference in measured expressive language age had increased from 3.5 months to 7.7 months. However, this gain score difference was not statistically significant; +

While none of these differences were statistically significant they emphasise the greater potential of the children of parents with higher mean PAAT total scores (>150) to achieve language gain scores. This in itself was considered to be reinforcing for these parents and as such they were more likely to be "more open, innovative and persistent" in contrast with the parents with lower mean PAAT total scores (<120) whose classification of being "defensive, uncertain and less persistent" was in itself reinforced by the minimum language gains achieved by their children.

The distinctive attitudes of the parents with high or low scores became even more apparent when the subset items were used as a basis for counselling parents during the language programme.

(vi) Items which differentiate between parents with high and low attitude scores.

Table 6.5 presents the PAAT subset mean scores for parents with high and low total PAAT scores. Table 6.6 presents items that markedly differentiated between the attitudes of parents with high and low scores on the PAAT.

There was no significant difference between the subset mean scores of parents with either high or low PAAT scores. + However, the different subset scores again emphasised the different attitudes of families to teaching their children. They demonstrated that the greatest difference was (i) in parents' attitude towards teaching (mean difference 11.6) and (ii) in the higher level of frustration (mean difference 8.5) expressed by parents with lower PAAT total scores.

The items in Table 6.6 illustrate items where a 60 per cent or more difference between the two parent groups occurred.

These items suggest areas that could be focused upon in a parent curriculum for families with a low prognosis for successful participation in an educational programme for their children. Parents with extremely low PAAT scores needed help in understanding just what was involved in teaching their children, and in maintaining interest in parent-child teaching and learning tasks.

+ Using Cochran and Cox's (1957) formula for testing the significance of the computed t when variances differ, as shown by an F-test.

TABLE 6.4

Characteristics of children whose parents
has either high (>150) or low (<120)
mean P A A T total scores at 0_2 ∅

	N	Mean PAAT Total Score	Mean Chron. age of children yrs mths	Average no. of children per family	Mean Stanford Binet I.Q. score	Mean RRLA at 0_1 months	Mean RRLA at 0_2 months	Mean RELA at 0_1 months	Mean RELA at 0_2 months
Parents with mean P A A T total <120	10	114.0	5 11	3	33.0	19.6	19.6	14.5	13.2
Parents with mean P A A T total >150	23	155.8	5 6	3	39.2	25.2	27.0	18.0	20.1

∅ 0_2 was the second observation point for standardised testing of the sample and occurred one year after the first standardised testing and commencement of the programme at observation point 0_1.

RRLA.   Reynell Receptive Language Age (Reynell 1969b).
RELA.   Reynell Expressive Language Age (Reynell 1969b).

TABLE 6.5

P A A T subset means and standard
deviations for parents with
high and low P A A T total scores

	N	Creativity		Control		Play		Teaching/ Learning		Frustration	
		X̄	S.D.	X̄	S.D.	X̄	S.D.	X̄	S.D.	X̄	S.D.
Parents with mean P A A T Total < 120	10	22.7	3.1	22.7	1.4	25.0	4.3	23.1	2.8	22.0	2.7
Parents with mean P A A T Total > 150	23	29.2	2.9	28.7	2.5	32.8	3.2	34.7	2.5	30.5	2.0

Attention to parent attitude, particularly those differences presented in Table 6.6, should, if possible, precede the introduction of teaching specific language or social skills. Furthermore, parent attitude needed to be monitored carefully during the programme as a constructive attitude proved to be such an important prerequisite for the acquisition and application of teaching skills.

(vii) **Limitations of using the PAAT with parents of intellectually handicapped children.**
    This was the first time the PAAT had been used with such a population and outside of the United States (see above Ch. 4, p. 69). As such, the interpretation of PAAT results, as an indication of the subjects' attitudes towards their handicapped children, need to be carefully examined.
    While the overall reliability of the instrument was high, an item analysis indicated a number of items with a negative or low correlation to the total PAAT scale. As shown in Table 6.7, seven PAAT items, three of them in the Creativity subset, correlated negatively with the total scale. These results may well reflect the behaviour modification techniques used in many training programmes for intellectually handicapped children (Tramontana 1971; Watson 1974), and in the structured language training programme developed for these children (see above Ch. 3, p. 57 and Appendix III). This finding is reflected in parent's attitudes towards the use of praise (Item 34) and reinforcement (Item 46). Item 36, regarding solitary play, would be expected to be answered negatively by parents of handicapped children because of memories of the historic neglect of such children. Parents were also disinclined to express uncertainty or to try to develop an ability in the child to forestall closure (Item 26 and 43). The items shown in Table 6.7 also had low mean scores.

Conclusion
    The Parent As A Teacher Inventory is a useful instrument, with some limitations, for understanding the child rearing expectations of parents of intellectually handicapped children. The total PAAT score of parents at either the upper or lower extremes served as an excellent guide for identifying those who would be most and least successful as teachers in a home-based child language training programme.
    Mothers and fathers who took part in this study made it clear that they did *not* want to be placated merely because they were parents of intellectually handicapped children. Although they expressed some reservations about their ability to succeed in teaching their children, they also demonstrated a willingness to learn how to develop language skills and monitor progress. After all, one hundred and two families stayed with the programme for three years.

TABLE 6.6

Selected P A A T Items differentiating
between high and low parent groups

	Item.	Group	% Desirable
1.	I get tired of all the questions my child asks.	High Low	92 30
9.	Playing with my child makes me feel restless.	High Low	96 30
10.	It is hard for me to tell when my child has learned something.	High Low	96 20
12.	I get tired of all the fears my child talks about.	High Low	100 40
13.	There are some things I just don't want my child to talk about.	High Low	82 20
20.	It is difficult for me to think of things to say to my child during play.	High Low	96 30
21.	When my child plays with toys, the pretending seems foolish.	High Low	100 40
28.	When at play with my child, I prefer games that have rules rather than the make-believe kind of play.	High Low	91 20
39.	It is difficult for me to stay interested when playing with my child.	High Low	82 30
41.	My child wants to play too long at one time.	High Low	87 0
45.	It is easy for me to use toys when teaching my child.	High Low	93 30
48.	It's allright for my child to have secrets from me.	High Low	83 10
50.	If we play whenever my child wants to, not much learning will take place.	High Low	83 10

Note: The "low" group of parents scored 120 or less on the P A A T and were less able to benefit from the Language Training Programme;

TABLE 6.7

Percentage desirable response for items at
issue for P A A T responses of 101 parents
of intellectually handicapped children.

Item and Desirable Response	R(total)	Mean	Desirable %	Undesirable %
Creativity Subset				
26. I want my child to have all of his questions ansered.	- .25	1.8	17	84
(No; willing to express uncertainty in answering child's questions).				
36. It is all right for my child to spend a lot of time playing alone.	- .17	2.3	43	58
(Yes; creative people often spend long periods in solitary pursuits).				
46. I seldom tell my child his work is good or bad so that my child can make up his own mind.	- .21	1.9	19	82
(Yes; lets child judge own work refrains from judging so that child judges work on the basis of its intrinsic merit).				
Frustration Subset				
42. When my child shows off I ignore it.	- .01	2.5	53	48

148

TABLE 6.7 (continued)

Item and Desirable Response	R(total)	Mean	Desirable %	Undesirable %
(No; pays attention to child's showing off).				
Control Subset				
23. While we play, my child should be the person in control.	- .18	2.5	54	47
(No; wants to share play dominance with child).				
43. I feel unhappy when I don't know an answer to my child's question.	- .03	2.4	58	43
(No; comfortable is not knowing all the answers to child's questions because s/he wants child to develop a questioning attitude).				
Play Subset				
34. I try to praise my child a lot when we play.	- .39	1.7	10	91
(No; recognises that the play process is rewarding in itself to child).				

149

The active participation of parents of intellectually handicapped children in language programmes should hopefully encourage a closer relationship between themselves and professionals working in the field. It can be shown that intervention programmes, such as the one in this study, have built up children's language skills. The involved parents also seemed to benefit in that their own feelings of frustration and helplessness were reduced.

It should not be inferred that home-based educational programmes will eliminate all the problems of atypical children, or resolve their parents' innermost conflicts and anxieties. Certainly the degree to which parental adjustment is influenced by having an intellectually handicapped child depends on many factors. However, one important variable appeared to be the opportunity to participate as members of a multidisciplinary team in an education programme designed to help their children. Another was the opportunity (that existed during the language intervention programme), for parents to focus on, and openly discuss, vital parent/child interaction variables.

The PAAT items have enabled parents in this programme to identify and examine attitude variables which were integral to successful teaching. Furthermore, scores on these items have helped identify those parents who would be most successful and those who would be least successful.

Chapter Seven

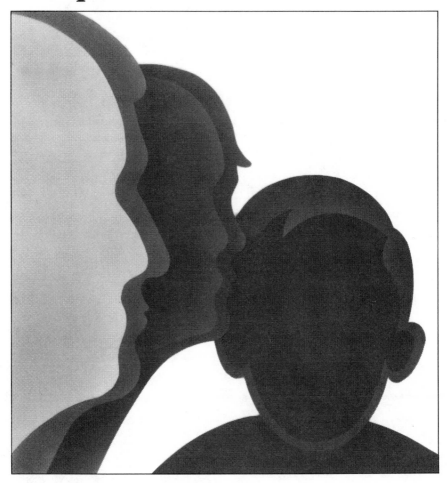

N=1 Case Studies

Preliminary Considerations.

The search for sources of variability within individuals and the use of $N = 1$ designs and teaching procedures may appear to be contrary to one of the most cherished goals of this study, that is the establishment of generality of findings. Identifying the sources of variability on different language tasks by particular subjects, however, should provide indications of possible sources of variability in other subjects being taught similar tasks. Therefore identifying sources of variability may be regarded as a primary technique for establishing generality. For example, if the five case studies below provide evidence of factors that contribute to variability in learning a language skill then this is likely to contribute to an understanding of how other subjects might learn such a skill.

These case studies are precise and controlled. Videotapes of home-based teaching and independent weekly probes (see Ch. 4, p. 70) have made it possible to present data which are also reliable. However, it is unrealistic to expect that a given variable, for example a parent's ability to cue a child, or to persevere with teaching will have the same effects on all similar intellectually handicapped subjects. These case studies demonstrate individual parents' skills, problems and achievements.

A problem that many parents raise is whether a controlled structured teaching situation can also be flexible. For example, if a particular teaching procedure works well in one case but works less well or fails when attempts are made to replicate this (see for example the comparison of case studies III and IV, p. 172) with other cases, can slight alterations be made? The case studies provide evidence of both variability in performance and demonstrate the opportunities for flexibility in teaching that exist. Functional analysis procedures allow for the examination of the effectiveness of a given procedure for a particular child. Consequently, when using functional analysis if the procedures are ineffective then they can be changed. For example, if alterations in teaching procedures or tasks do not produce improvement in the relevant language skills then differences in the child's background, his/her personality characteristics, home setting, or particular difficulties pertaining to his/her particular condition of intellectual handicap can be noted and other procedures substituted. These observations then form the basis for procedural changes which can be trialled with this child or type of child at a later date. The controlled structured teaching and recording in these case studies provide evidence of variability and of the opportunities for flexibility. In turn, conclusions about generalisation of language skills can be made.

CASE STUDY I

Responding to simple commands. Naming some objects in every day use.

The subject is a 35 month old Down's syndrome girl*, the second of two children. The child "Kay" was in the Target Teaching Group from 0_2 to 0_5 (see above Ch. 3, p. 58). Kay was assessed on the criterion language tasks at 0_2 (Ch. 3, p. 58). As a result of this assessment, the receptive and expressive language tasks that Kay's parents set out to teach are those presented below. (Receptive Language Tasks i to vi inclusive and Expressive Language Tasks iii and iv.).

Deciding what to Teach.

When the receptive and expressive language tasks baseline was drawn at 0_2 (see Fig. 3.1 and Appendix V). Kay had successfully responded to **four** of the ten items in Receptive Language Task No. I and had satisfactorily mastered the Expressive Language Tasks I and II. For example, in the Receptive Language Task No. 1 Kay satisfactorily performed the following

---

* 35 months old at 0_2.

actions in response to verbal commands from her mother. The verbal commands were (i) "Come Here!", (ii) "Show Me!", (iii) "Wave Bye-Bye!" and (iv) "Sit Down!". Satisfactory is defined as performing the action correctly on **four** out of five occasions when the presentation of the stimulus commands had been randomised. Kay had not achieved criterion in any of the **receptive** language tasks and therefore her family began teaching her at Receptive Language Task I. Kay had achieved criterion at 0_2 on Expressive Language Tasks I and II (see Appendix II) and therefore expressive language teaching began with Expressive Language Task III.

Kay's Mother's Teaching Skills

At the commencement of the teaching programme, Kay's mother ably demonstrated the ability to get Kay to look at and attend to the task at hand. She worked close to Kay, skillfully using attention getting techniques (as indicated in the preparatory section of the language manual, see above Ch. 3 and Appendix II). Kay's mother did not commence teaching in any session until Kay was following the mother with her eyes. She rewarded Kay with enthusiastic praise **immediately** following a satisfactory response.

Receptive Language Tasks mastered by Kay during the period of teaching 0_2 and 0_5 (see above Fig. 3.1 and below Fig. 7.1).

The receptive language tasks set out below were if appropriate first taught as behaviours to be imitated, and then as actions to be performed in response to verbal commands. Details of the teaching strategies used are those set out in the language manual (Appendix III). The Receptive Language Tasks I to VI are those which Kay mastered during the nine months of her mother's teaching. The Receptive Language Tasks I to VI were as follows (see also Fig. 7.1).

Receptive Language Task I (R.L.I.)
Responding to stimulus verbal commands.

(i) **Come** Here	(ii) **Show** Me	(iii) **Wave** Bye-Bye
(iv) **Sit Down**	(v) **Stand** Up	(vi) **Lie Down**
(vii) **Open** the Door	(viii) **Shut** the Door	(ix) **Stay There**
(x) **Don't Touch**		

Receptive Language Task II (R.L.II)
Responding to stimulus verbal commands by correctly imitating the response.

(i) **Turn** off the light	(ii) **Fold** your arms	(iii) **Comb** your hair
(iv) **Brush** your teeth	(v) **Wipe** your nose	(vi) **Close** your eyes
(vii) **Open** your eyes	(viii) **Wash** your face	(ix) **Wash** your ears
(x) **Brush** your shoes		

Receptive Language Task III (R.L.III)
Pointing to objects named.

(i) Show me the **keys**	(ii) Show me the **ball**	(iii) Show me the **baby** doll
(iv) Show me the **bell**	(v) Show me the **car**	(vi) Show me the **comb**
(vii) Show me the **hat**	(viii) Show me the **shoe**	(ix) Show me the **cup**
(x) Show me the **plate**		

Receptive Language Task IV (R.L.IV)

(i) Show me the **bread**	(ii) Show me the **butter**	(iii) Show me the **fork**
(iv) Show me the **knife**	(v) Show me the **hammer**	(vi) Show me the **nail**
(vii) Show me the **paper**	(viii) Show me the **spoon**	(ix) Show me the **towel**
(x) Show me the **water**		

In tasks III and IV the child is required to **point** to the object named by the parent or teacher. For the task to be mastered the child is required to point to the correct item in the presence of any **two** others.

154

Receptive Language Task V (R.L.V)

Using of objects that the child can point to.

(i) **Turn** the keys	(ii) **Throw** the ball	(iii) **Put on** the hat
(iv) **Comb** your hair	(v) **Wash** your face	(vi) **Ring** the bell
(vii) **Push** the car	(viii) **Make** the bed	

The child is expected to **imitate** or perform the correct action on command.

Dolls and other toys should be used when teaching. Note that tasks here may involve repeating tasks previously mastered in Receptive Language Task II.

Receptive Language Task VI (R.L.VI)

Looking for and finding concealed objects.

Objects: e.g. Ball, car, comb, shoe, cup, fork, knife, hammer. The child will have learned to point to objects named when **three** objects are placed in front of him or her. As many as eight objects are spread on a table but are concealed under a cloth. The parent shows the child the objects and then covers them. The stimulus command is "FIND THE ..." The child is required to lift the cloth and to point to the item named.

Weekly Record

The weekly graphical record of Kay's number of correct responses for receptive and expressive language tasks is shown below in Fig. 7.1. Independent assessment took place each week on the particular receptive and expressive tasks being taught to Kay (see above Ch. 4, Assessment procedures). As soon as criterion had been achieved in a given task then Kay's mother was advised to begin teaching the next task. For example, criterion in Receptive Language Task I involves ten correct responses out of ten, when the presentation of items is randomised. Kay achieved criterion at the end of the third week in Receptive Language Task I. Table 7.1 illustrates the number of teaching sessions as well as the number of weeks required for each receptive language task.

FIG. 7.1

Weekly Graphical Record of Kay's correct responses for receptive and expressive language tasks O_2 to O_5

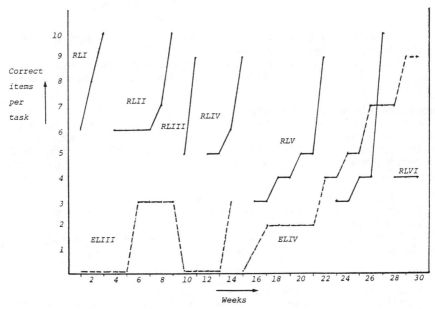

155

The graph of weekly responses to Receptive Language Task I (Fig. 7.1) shows Kay accomplishing six tasks at the end of the first week, and going on to criterion of ten at the end of the third week. These **weekly** checks of Kay's receptive language responses may also be regarded as **retention** tests. The positive social reinforcement contingency required that the independent tester make immediate judgements about the correctness of the response. The criteria in the programme also required that the tester keep a record of correct responses so that the mother could be advised as to when to change to a different task. Videotapes were made of a selected number of training sessions.*

TABLE 7.1

Number of Teaching Sessions and Number of weeks required for each <u>receptive</u> language task by Kay before <u>criterion</u> in each task was achieved.

Receptive Language Tasks	No. of Teaching Sessions**	No. of Weeks per Task
I	30	3
I I	60	6
I I I	20	2
I V	40	4
V	70	7
I V	50	5

The **minimum** of teaching sessions is recorded here. This is based on parental advice of two ten minute sessions per day, five days a week.**

Records do illustrate parents practising more than a minimum of two hours direct teaching per week but two ten minute parent teaching sessions per day, five days a week is also considered to be just what most parents can possibly sustain.

Daily Teaching of Receptive Language

A random number of daily teaching sessions were videotaped* and records of subjects' responses were collected. Kay was one of the subjects for which daily teaching records of particular language tasks were collected. The description which follows describes the **daily** teaching of Receptive Language Task number I (see Fig. 7.2) and Expressive Language Task II (see Fig. 7.3).

Receptive Language Task I (Responses to Commands)

The ten commands or simple verbal directions for teaching and rehearsing in Receptive Language Task I are as follows:
- (i) Come Here
- (ii) Show Me
- (iii) Wave Bye-Bye
- (iv) Sit Down
- (v) Stand Up
- (vi) Lie Down

---

* Videotape used: High Density J Standard Sony AV 34/20: Portapack.
** Recorded Daily Teaching Sessions — Two ten minute sessions per day, five days a week.

156

(vii) Open the Door   (viii) Shut the Door   (ix) Stay There
(x) Don't Touch

Each stimulus command was presented separately by Kay's mother. The description of the teaching of each **separate** stimulus command is as follows:

Stimulus Command I "Come Here!" (S.C. I)

Kay was instructed to watch her mother, to listen to the command and then to respond. Correct responses were **immediately** followed by enthusiastic praise from her mother. This was definitely a strong point of Kay's mother's teaching. No response or incorrect response received **no** verbal praise from Kay's mother, but was generally followed by "Let's do that again!" The criterion for each presentation of the stimulus command was four correct responses in any five presentations (see Fig. 7.2). When Kay had correctly responded on four out of five occasions then her mother moved on to the next command. This home-based training situation may be presented diagramatically as:

$$S^1 \quad R \quad S^{R+}$$

(i) S^1 represents the command stimulus
(ii) R represents the correct response
(iii) S^{R+} represents the positive social reinforcer.

All correct responses were reinforced so that the graph (Fig. 7.2) showing the number of correct responses in any five presentations of the stimulus command, represents the $S^1/R/S^{R+}$ model presented above.

In the five sessions (five stimulus commands presented per session) Kay demonstrated correct responses (four out of five) on four of the training sessions. The teaching procedure carried out by Kay's mother was as follows:

(i) Mother placed the child on the floor some three to four paces away, and then issued the command "Come Here!" — or alternatively, the mother placed herself three to four paces from the child, and when she had gained the child's attention, issued the command "Come Here!"

(ii) Kay responded by crawling or walking to the mother.

(iii) The mother enthusiastically praised the child — "Well done, Kay!", "Good Kay," "What a clever girl!" — looking directly at the child, often holding her hands as she praised her daughter.

Stimulus Command II "Show Me!" (S.C. II)

S.C. II (Fig 7.2) shows the number of correct responses for each teaching presentation of five stimulus commands per session. Kay was observed during seven teaching sessions (35 presentations of the stimulus command) and achieved criterion of four out of five correct responses during the last four teaching sessions. The teaching procedure was as follows:

(i) Mother placed one toy (a teddy bear) within Kay's reach and then issued the command, "Show me Teddy!"

(ii) The child responded by looking at and by picking up Teddy or by pointing to Teddy. (In the pre-training sessions mother had taken Kay's hand and, following the command "Show me Teddy!" had placed the child's hand on the Teddy bear and then followed this with enthusiastic praise).

(iii) Kay's mother enthusiastically praised the child as above.

Stimulus Command III "Wave Bye-Bye!" (S.C. III)

Criterion was achieved in all teaching sessions. (20 presentations of the stimulus command). Through the process of successive approximation (reinforcement of behaviours which approximate a correct response to the command "Wave Bye-Bye!") and physical help, Kay's family had taught and rehearsed this behaviour from the time Kay was able to attend and respond to the command, "Wave Bye-Bye!" **Modelling** by the mother and other members of the family was the strategy the family had used to successfully teach this command.

Stimulus Command IV "Sit Down!" (S.C. IV)

Criterion was achieved on the third, fourth and fifth training sessions. The procedure was as follows:

(i) Mother decided that Kay should learn to sit down herself rather than demonstrate the behaviour with a doll. Mother demonstrated the behaviour by sitting down on the carpeted floor upon the command "Sit Down!", and made Kay do the same.

(ii) Observable training sessions occurred without mother sitting down. Mother looked at the child and then said: "Kay sit down!", or "sit down, Kay!"

(iii) Kay responded by sitting down on the carpeted floor. On the three occasions in the first session, and the one occasion during the second session when there was no response, or an incorrect response, Kay either turned away and pretended not to hear, or indeed walked away to do something else, Kay's mother made no response to this incorrect behaviour. Mother enthusiastically praised Kay — "Well done, Kay!", "Good Kay." "What a clever girl!" — always looking directly at Kay when Kay responded correctly.

Stimulus Command V "Stand Up!" (S.C. V)

Criterion was achieved in the sixth, seventh and eighth training sessions (see Fig. 7.2). Kay early showed an understanding of the command, "Stand Up!", by demonstrating the behaviour with a doll. However, her mother insisted that Kay perform the behaviour herself, even though when Kay was placed on the floor there was every likelihood that Kay would roll around and not attend to the stimulus command.

Preparation for getting Kay to stand up.

(i) Mother and Kay would sit together on the carpeted floor — mother would say "Stand Up!" and, holding Kay's hand, would stand up, pulling Kay with her. This was done on some ten occasions prior to the recorded training session in which Kay had to stand up **without** her mother's assistance.

(ii) Mother placed Kay on the floor with a dining-room chair alongside to help Kay pull herself up if necessary. Kay's mother placed herself close to Kay, looked at her and said "Stand Up!" giving non-verbal demonstrations and enouragement with her hands.

(iii) Kay responded by hauling herself to her feet. On the occasions during the first five training sessions when Kay failed to respond or responded incorrectly, (see Fig. 7.2), she invariably rolled on the floor or crawled away. Kay's mother reinforced each of Kay's **correct** responses with enthusiastic verbal praise. Incorrect responses were either ignored, or Kay was picked up and placed back in the original position. Whenever the situation became stressful for Kay her mother responded by cuddling her. The close proximity of Kay's mother to her and the likelihood of success reduced stress for Kay to a minimum.

Stimulus Command VI "Lie Down!" (S.C. VI)

This particular activity was easily mastered in the home setting. The amount of movement from a sitting to a lying down position was relatively minimal. This command had been used regularly by her family when Kay had been put to bed, and in the recorded session with Kay, her mother demonstrated Kay's correct response to this command.

Stimulus Command VII "Open the Door!" (S.C. VII)

Criterion was achieved at the third training session. For this task the door on a doll's house was used. A similar doll's house door was used at the health clinic for the testing sessions. The teaching procedure was as follows:

(i) Baseline testing established that Kay only intermittently understood the command. Her mother **demonstrated** the response to this command by saying "Open the door, Mummy!" and then proceeded to open the doll's house door when Kay was attending. This was followed by Kay being physically guided to "open the door". As soon as mother and the teacher felt that Kay definitely understood the command, the recorded teaching took place over seven sessions (see Fig. 7.2).

(ii) During the first ten recorded responses Kay made six incorrect responses (see Fig. 7.2 S.C. VII) — ignoring the command twice, pointing to a window, pointing to the house generally, pointing to the roof twice. Criterion responses were recorded during the remaining training sessions. There is certainly much evidence that Kay's mother rehearsed the activities between observed recording sessions, and certainly between the second and third recorded session. However, this must always be allowed for and expected in any home based teaching programme.

(iii) **Incorrect** responses were ignored by Kay's mother, or she responded by saying "No Kay, try again", "Open the door!" It did appear that incorrect responses may have occurred in the earlier sessions because the non-verbal cue of Kay's mother looking directly at the door when she said "Open the door!" was omitted. This need for **very clear** non verbal cues was discussed with Kay's mother. Correct responses were as usual enthusiastically praised by Kay's mother.

Stimulus Command VIII "Shut the Door!" (S.C. VIII)

The same teaching procedure was followed as for stimulus command "Open the door!" Much confusion occured in early training and only on the sixth session was criterion achieved. There is a definite need here for these two tasks to be taught together so that the stimulus commands become "Open the door, now, shut the door!" This **clarification** of the stimulus command took place in the sixth and seventh training sessions and criterion was then achieved (see Fig. 7.2).

Stimulus Command IX "Stay There!" (S.C. IX)

This stimulus command required Kay to stay in position and not follow the mother when she moved away, either from the dining room table or from a position in which mother and Kay were sitting together. It was emphasised throughout that this activity in particular should be played as a **game**, though it also represented Kay's ability to do what she was told. To make the activity clear, Kay's mother placed a cushion on the floor, or taped the outline of a circle with plastic tape on the floor and then, after placing Kay in the circle, issued the command "Stay there!" It needs to be stressed that whether or not Kay stayed in position clearly depended on whether she was easily distracted. There were, in fact, ten training sessions before Kay achieved criterion. Fifteen observed training sessions took place overall, though again, Kay's mother indicated that this game was also played on many occasions during the first three weeks when Kay and her mother were practising Receptive Language Task I (see Fig. 7.2).

Stimulus Command X "Don't Touch!" (S.C. X)

This activity was not new to Kay, though she had failed the task when the baseline testing took place. Criterion with her mother was achieved on the fourth teaching session. The teaching procedure was as follows:

Kay's mother placed a toy or object in front of Kay who was immediately attracted to pick it up — mother looked sternly at Kay and with raised forefinger said briskly "Don't touch!" As soon as Kay declined to touch it mother said "Good, Kay. Well done. Now you can pick it up." Kay had only momentarily to decline upon the stimulus command "Don't touch!" for a correct response to be recorded. This "momentary" response latency required for a correct response, was considered realistic in that this would allow Kay's mother time between saying "Don't touch!" and removing her child from a potentially dangerous or unacceptable situation.

Expressive Language Tasks mastered by Kay during the period of teaching 0_2 to 0_5 (See Fig. 3.1).

When Kay's expressive language profile was assessed at 0_2 Kay could successfully imitate four sounds as required in Expressive Language Tasks I and II (see Appendix II and Appendix III). Kay therefore began her expressive language exercises with the naming of body parts task (Expressive Language Task III). Mastery of these tasks is considered to have been achieved when the subject can successfully name **six** out of eight body parts. It is stressed in this and other expressive language tasks that any approximation to the correct response that the child utters should be reinforced (rewarded) provided the parent or teacher is able to discriminate among the different responses being made. When weekly criterion testing took place, then any approxima-

FIG. 7.2

Sessional Graphical Record of Kay's correct
responses for Receptive Language Task I

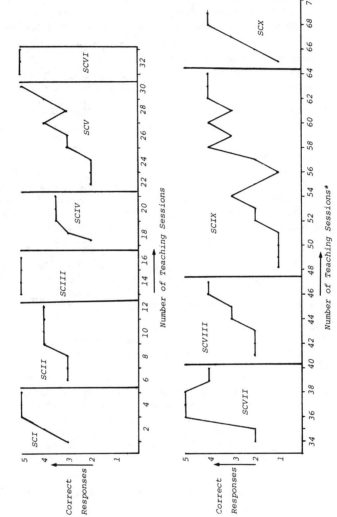

* Each recorded session lasts approximately 10 minutes and involves five presentations
  of each stimulus command.

160

tion to a correct response was also counted as correct, provided the tester was able to understand the utterance being made and that it could be discriminated from other utterances. Only one specific expressive language task was assessed each week. Table 7.2 below illustrates the number of training sessions and the number of weeks required for each expressive language task for Kay. After fourteen weeks of teaching, Kay did not achieve criterion in Expressive Language Task III (see Fig. 7.1). From the fifteenth week Kay's ability to successfully name objects (Expressive Language Task IV) was taught and assessed. It should be noted that during the fourteen weeks of teaching Kay to name body parts, other relevant exercises could also be practised, though it was always emphasised to Kay's mother as to which task was being assessed each week. Wherever possible, there is maximum correspondence between the receptive and expressive tasks in the manual (see Appendix III) particularly as related to the sequence of tasks. However, it does appear that for Kay (and indeed for many other children), the expressive language task "Naming of body parts" comes much too early in the sequence (see Appendix II).

TABLE 7.2

Number of Teaching Sessions and Number of Weeks required for each Expressive Language Task by Kay before criterion on each task was achieved or before Kay was assessed on another task.

Expressive Language Task	No. of Teaching Sessions*	No. of Weeks per Task
III Naming of Body Parts	140	14
IV Naming of Objects	184	15

* Two ten minute sessions, five days per week, is considered to be the minimum number of parent teaching sessions for each expressive language task, though in practice much more "teaching" may occur incidentally in daily interaction.

Expressive Language Teaching (Expressive Language Task IV)

Regular evaluation of Expressive Language Task IV, the naming of objects, commenced in the fifteenth week of Stage II (see Figs. 7.1 and 7.3). Kay had failed to score at all on Expressive Language Task III and Expressive Language Task IV when her expressive language profile was drawn at 0_2 (see Fig. 3.1 and Appendix V). Kay's mother had commenced teaching Expressive Language Task III and Kay had been assessed on this task for fourteen weeks (see Fig. 7.1). However, apart from results achieved in weeks 6, 7, 8, 9, and 13, there was much indication that Kay was having great difficulty with this task and therefore she was switched on the fifteenth week to being taught and assessed on Expressive Language Task IV, the naming of objects. During the previous fourteen weeks, Kay's expressive language performance was always assessed on Expressive Language Task III, the naming of body parts. However, at no time was it specified that this task was to be taught to the exclusion of any others (only that this was the task being assessed), and there was every opportunity for Kay's mother or father also to teach the naming of objects exercises, Expressive Language Task IV and V (see Appendix II and Appendix III).

There is much evidence in the literature of correspondence between receptive and expressive language tasks and that the first words children utter usually make reference to particular objects or persons (Bloom 1973, and Clarke 1973). This ability to say words is generally helped by the child's comprehension of the object and this comprehension depends in turn on the many situations in which the child has experienced an association between an

161

acoustic event, (Kay's mother saying the word "ball") and the object. There is in the language manual (see Appendix III) a close relationship generally between receptive and expressive language tasks.

Fifteen weeks to teach the ability to name objects (Expressive Language Task IV)

Fig. 7.3 and Table 7.2 indicate the number of teaching sessions that were required to achieve criterion in this task. Each recorded session involves five presentations of the stimulus command. Each individual graph in Fig. 7.3 indicates the number of correct responses per presentation, and the total number of recorded presentations. Criterion in any training session is achieved by a recording of four correct responses in any five presentations. For example, in S.R.1 ("Say Ball!"), criterion was achieved in the fifteenth, seventeenth, eighteenth, nineteenth and twentieth training sessions (see Fig. 7.3). Therefore, by the time S.R.II was being assessed, Kay had already experienced one hundred presentations of the command "Say Ball!"

The expressive language stimulus responses the child was required to utter were:

S.R.I	"BALL"	S.R.II	"BABY"	S.R.III	"KEYS"
S.R.IV	"BELL"	S.R.V	"CAR"	S.R.VI	"COMB"
S.R.VII	"HAT"	S.R.VIII	"SHOE"	S.R.IX	"CUP"
S.R.X	"MILK"				

FIG. 7.3

Sessional Graphical Record of Kay's
correct responses for Expressive Language
Task IV (naming of objects)

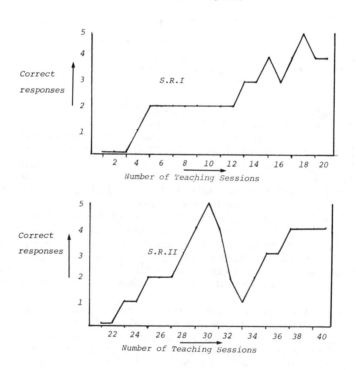

162

FIG. 7.3 (continued)

Sessional Graphical Record of Kay's
correct responses for Expressive Language
Task IV (naming of objects)

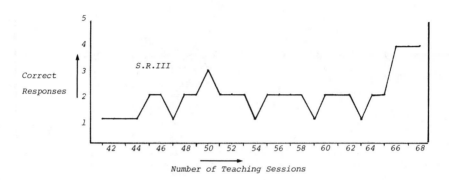

Number of Teaching Sessions

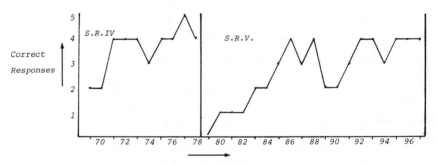

Number of Teaching Sessions

163

FIG. 7.3 (continued)

Sessional Graphical Record of Kay's
correct responses for Expressive Language
Task IV (naming of objects)

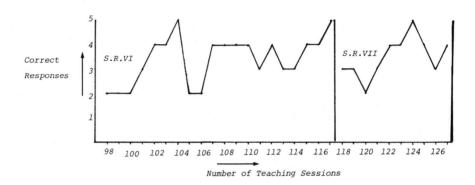

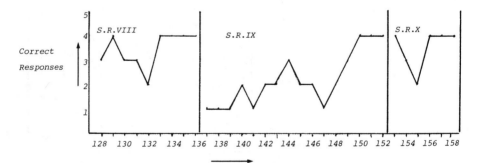

In each of these expressive language exercises Kay's mother was taught and advised to use vocal imitation as a prompting device. For example, Kay's mother could back up the question "What is this?" with the command "Say ball!" Kay's mother gradually faded the imitative prompt and always reinforced successive approximations to the desired response. As long as Kay's mother could satisfactorily discriminate Kay's vocal response, then this was not only reinforced but scored as a correct response. This pattern of teaching applies to the ten stimulus commands in Expressive Language Task IV. The results (Table 7.3) illustrate that Kay required the following number of training sessions and presentations of the stimulus command before being considered able to respond satisfactorily and therefore successfully complete Expressive Language Task IV.

TABLE 7.3

Number of Teaching Sessions and Presentations
required for Expressive Language Task IV
for subject Kay to achieve criterion on
each task.

S.C.	S.R.	No. of Teaching Sessions	No. of Presentations
I	BALL	20	100
II	BABY	20	100
III	KEYS	30	150
IV	BELL	10	50
V	CAR	20	100
VI	COMB	20	100
VII	HAT	10	50
VIII	SHOE	9	45
IX	CUP	20	100
X	MILK	7	35

Conclusion

Kay's mother has proved to be a most effective teacher in that she has demonstrated an ability to shape and reinforce Kay in the teaching situation. Moreover, Kay not only achieved criterion on six receptive language tasks (R.L.I to R.L.VI inclusive, see Appendix II) and on one expressive language task (E.L.IV, see Appendix II), but the acquisition of these language skills

TABLE 7.4

Kay's Reynell Developmental Language Age
Scores in Months.

	0_1	0_2	0_3	0_4	0_5	0_6
Receptive Language Age	05*	05	18	19	20	28
Expressive Language Age	05	05	20	20	16	29
Chronological Age	23	35	38	41	44	56

* 05 months was the language age recorded wherever a child failed to reach the minimum language age score on the Reynell Language Test (Reynell 1969b) of 06 months.

165

appears to have generalised and been retained as indicated by the specific language age scores achieved by Kay during the thirty-three months of the programme (see Table 7.4).

The conclusions to be drawn from this data and from Kay's language behaviour at the end of the programme are as follows:

(i) That Kay's receptive language ability improved remarkably during the first three months of the teaching programme O_2 to O_3 (a gain score of thirteen months in three months) and thereafter plateaued. However, the initial gain score was not lost and this improvement in receptive language ability continued in the year following the specific treatment programme (O_5 to O_6). This continued gain is largely due to Kay's mother's effectiveness as a teacher and to her ability to sustain that teaching in Stage III (see Fig. 3.1) with minimal support. However, it should be noted that the discrepancy between Kay's receptive language age and chronological age from O_4 to O_6 is beginning to widen. Also, it seems unlikely that Kay would have achieved this level of receptive language skill had it not been for the marked gain score achieved and maintained during the nine months of the teaching programme. Certainly, the discrepancy between the receptive language age and chronological age was greatest at O_2 (see Fig. 3.1) **before** the commencement of specific teaching.

(ii) Kay's expressive language age improved remarkably (gain score of fifteen months in three months) in the first three months of teaching (O_2 to O_3), was maintained until O_4 (see Fig. 3.1) but slipped back at O_5 (see Table 7.4). However, Kay did achieve a gain score of eleven months in nine months from O_2 to O_5 and achieved a gain of thirteen months in the following twelve months (O_5 to O_6). In Kay's case the speech therapist reported improved articulation at O_6 due largely to Kay's mother's persistence and " . . . the resulting motivation developed in Kay". Kay's mother is aware that Kay, like other Down's syndrome children, is organically capable of accurate articulation, and that this improvement often depends on motivation.

There is every indication in Kay's case that her overall language proficiency will continue to improve. Furthermore, the level of her expressive language **and** articulation at age four years eight months demonstrates a degree of progress which is due to **both** her mother's skill as a teacher and Kay's definite potential for greater language proficiency.

CASE STUDY II

(i) Responding to commands related to body space awareness.
(ii) Vocalising three imitative speech sounds.

The subject is a 5 years 1 month old* girl who had been variously diagnosed as brain damaged with some autistic characteristics. The child Amanda, was in the Target Teaching Group A from O_2 to O_5 (see above Ch. 3, p. 58). Amanda was assessed on the criterion language tasks at O_2 (see Ch. 3). As a result of this assessment the receptive and expressive language tasks that Amanda's parents set out to teach were those presented below. (see also Fig. 7.4).

Initial Diagnosis and evidence from parents (see above Ch. 3, p. 55)

When Amanda was first examined, there was little evidence that she could vocalise intelligibly, or that she played with other children. Her speech included some unintelligible vocalisations, though Amanda's mother indicated that on many occasions there were "long periods of total silence". Furthermore, the little speech that was intelligible was generally inappropriate to the situation and often echolalic in character. Amanda's parents and teachers reported that generally she was unresponsive to adult verbalisations and there was no evidence that Amanda could imitate modelled sounds. There were, however, examples that Amanda could respond to requests provided the cues were clear and provided they were supported by physical prompts.

---

* Amanda was 5 years 1 month at the commencement of teaching at O_2.

Receptive Language Tasks mastered by Amanda during the period of teaching 0_2 to 0_5 (see above Fig. 3.1).

The receptive Language Tasks indicated below are those **successfully** completed by Amanda during the teaching periods. The aim is for these language tasks to be sequential. However, where tasks appear difficult for a particular child then other tasks may be substituted, hence the apparent jump by Amanda from task IV to task XIV. Since Amanda's parents were regularly consulted on the tasks to be taught, they advised that Amanda should switch from task IV to task XIV as these were tasks on which Amanda was more likely to succeed.

Receptive Language Task IV (R.L. IV)
Pointing to objects named (as for Case Study 1, see above p. 154)

Receptive Language Task XIV (R.L. XIV)
Colour sorting task. Pointing to a named coloured cube when **three** different coloured cubes are presented.

Receptive Language Task XV (R.L. XV)
Commands and body/space awareness. Commands:
(i) Get **in** the box   (ii) Look **up**   (iii) Look **down**
(iv) Fall **down**   (v) Stand **up**   (vi) Sit **down**
(vii) Turn **round** and **round** (viii) Get **in** the circle
(ix) Walk **on** the line   (x) Crawl **under** the table

Receptive Language Task XVI (R.L. XVI)
Noun Vocabulary Group II (Rehearsal Task) Pointing to objects names (as for R.L. Task IV, see above Case Study I pages   ).

Receptive Language Task XVII (R.L. XVII)
Sorting exercise — concept big/little — criterion 80 per cent correct on a sort which involves 10 big items and 10 little items (see Appendix II).

Receptive Language Task XVIII (R.L. XVIII)
Pointing to colour named. Pointing to a named coloured cube when six different coloured cubes are presented.

Receptive Language Task XIX (R.L. XIX)
Commands involving verb and noun: responding to stimulus verbal commands:
(i) **Tear** the paper   (ii) **Draw** a line   (iii) **Draw** a circle
(iv) **Make** a tower (four or (v) **Ring** the bell   (vi) **Push** the car
      five blocks)

Receptive Language Task XV: Commands and Body-Space Awareness
Fig. 7.4 illustrates that Amanda achieved criterion on this task after seven weeks of teaching (weeks 8 to 15 inclusive), and after a minimum of sixty-six recorded teaching sessions. This particular teaching programme demonstrated that Amanda could be trained to comply with simple instructions. Since receptive language skills are important for any child to acquire in terms of their usefulness in daily living, the teaching method developed and analysed here was aimed to teach generalised instruction-following to prepositional requests. Fig. 7.5 indicates the number[σ] of teaching sessions required to teach these skills and the number of correct responses per session. It needs to be stressed that all these activities were presented as games to be played between Amanda and her family.

Method
The categories of prepositional requests are outlined above (Receptive Language Task XV — see also Appendices II and III). In these sessions allowance was made for teaching by

---

[σ] These represent the recorded teaching sessions, but Amanda's parents made it clear that they did practise these tasks on other occasions.

FIG. 7.4

Weekly graphical record of Amanda's correct
responses for Receptive and Expressive Language
Tasks 0_2 - 0_5

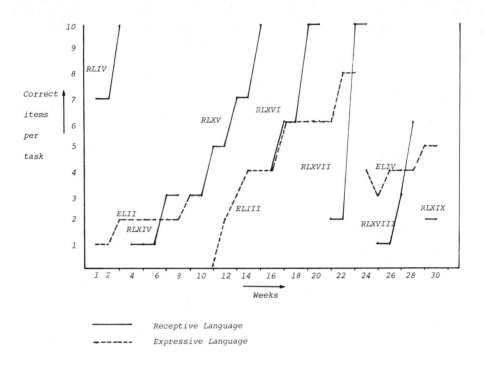

Correct items per task

Weeks

——————— Receptive Language

- - - - - - - Expressive Language

Amanda's mother prior to the session being recorded. Therefore, those sessions that have been recorded (as indicated below in Fig. 7.5) do not necessarily represent the total amount of teaching given to Amanda. In the recorded teaching sessions, five presentations of the stimulus command are presented on each occasion. These sessions took place daily in Amanda's home, in the family dining room, or once a week, under supervision by a trained teacher, in a room in a local health centre.

In the recorded teaching sessions the stimulus commands were presented to Amanda. If Amanda responded correctly, she was praised and given a raisin or, as with the expressive language task outlined below, on occasions a small amount of icecream. If Amanda made no response within 10 seconds of the presentation of the stimulus command then her mother would prompt her by physically guiding her through the response (getting **into** the carboard box on the floor, sitting **down**, turning **round** and **round**, crawling **under** the table, walking **on** the tape line on the floor) and immediately delivered praise and the raisin or icecream. An incorrect response usually produced "No . . . Amanda . . . do it this way" . . . then the request was presented again and Amanda would be prompted for the correct response, which was followed by praise "Good girl Amanda . . . well done Amanda" and the raisin or icecream. Physical prompts were faded out over many teaching sessions by gradually reducing the physical dimensions of the prompts until Amanda was responding correctly to the verbal requests without assistance. The teaching procedure continued for each separate command until Amanda reached a criterion of at least four out of five successive correct responses per session without prompting. If criterion was not reached in a session then teaching on the same receptive item was continued in the next session.

168

Testing Sessions

As indicated above, testing took place each week by an independent tester known to Amanda. (The results of these testing sessions are shown in Fig. 7.4). In these testing or probe sessions the trained requests were randomly interspersed with the untrained commands, beginning with Stimulus Command I "Get in the box" and moving through progressively to Stimulus Command X "Crawl under the table". As new commands were taught, they, along with previously taught commands, were interspersed during the testing session. The stimulus commands were **presented** in testing sessions as in the teaching sessions but responses were **never** prompted or followed by praise and the raisin or icecream; they were merely recorded by the tester. This does contrast with the recorded teaching session at home where all correct responses were reinforced.

Results

The graphs Fig. 7.5 show Amanda's performance during the daily recorded teaching sessions. The number of correct responses per session is determined by the correct response being made within 10 seconds.* Those commands that gave most difficulty were: I "Get in the box" — 45 presentations of the stimulus command; VII "Turn **round** and **round**" — 45

FIG. 7.5

Sessional graphical record of Amanda's correct* responses for Receptive Language task XV

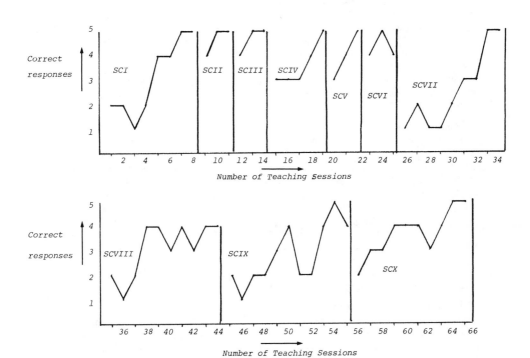

* The response latency of 10 seconds is important for these tasks as inability to respond correctly within 10 seconds was counted as a failure.
* Videotape used: High Density J Standard Sony AV 34/20: Portapack.

169

presentations of the stimulus command; VIII "Get in the circle" — 150 presentations of the stimulus command; IX "Walk on the line" — 55 presentations of the stimulus command; X "Crawl under the table" — 50 presentations of the stimulus command.

Expressive Language Teaching (Expressive Language Task II)

Daily probes of Amanda's attempts to imitate **correctly** three distinct sounds took place during the first ten weeks of the programme (see Expressive Language Task II, Fig. 7.4). Teaching sessions took place at home (generally across the dining room table) and once a week in a 2m x 2m room which contained a table and two chairs. In both settings the amount of external noise was minimal. Prior to the first session Amanda's parents agreed to try and reward any of Amanda's correct utterances by means of food such as raisins or potato crisps, or, indeed on occasions, with a lick of icecream, as well as rewarding her with much praise.

Recording Amanda's verbal utterances

Amanda's verbal utterances were tallied by a trained observer and random sessions in the home were videotaped.* During baseline sessions no attempt was made by the teacher to reinforce Amanda's verbal behaviour. During this time Amanda did not emit any vocalisations, either spontaneously or imitatively, and she failed to respond to simple verbal directions such as "Sit down", even though, when the baseline was drawn at 0_2, her teachers had recorded that she had achieved criterion in these receptive language tasks. Amanda emitted no vocalisations during baseline, so it was not possible at that time to bring her into contact with the reinforcer by reinforcing vocalisation. Therefore the imitation paradigm (as outlined in Appendix III) was chosen for teaching. This paradigm provides an opportunity to establish the contingencies by starting with other motor imitations **before** trying to attain vocal imitation. It is easier to train motor imitation than vocal imitation because the parent can manually move the child's arm through the required motion while the child sits still, and at the completion of the movement the parent can present the child with a reinforcer. In this procedure the manual prompts are continued by the teacher/parent. As Amanda began to acquire the motor behaviour then the prompts were gradually faded. Finally, the physical prompts were removed entirely because when Amanda could imitate a movement without a prompt (as in receptive language exercise IV — Pointing to objects named (see Appendix III)) — then the teacher was able to establish with her parents that the contingency had been established.

Motor Imitation before Vocal Imitation

In the initial phase of this ten week programme Amanda received training in hand movements prior to receiving direct "imitative vocal training". This was done because it was a readily trained behaviour which could be used to establish positive reinforcers and make the contingencies explicit for Amanda. When, therefore, Amanda emitted a current vocal response, the teacher or her mother would smile and say "Good Girl" and then present her with a raisin, or, in some instances, the lick of icecream. Within two weeks, under this teaching situation, Amanda had acquired vocal imitations, though the independent weekly record (see Fig. 7.4) indicates that only **one** sound was correctly imitated and that no sequence had been achieved until the third week (thirtieth teaching session**). However, at the end of the first two weeks, which involved twenty ten-minute teaching sessions, the motor imitation had accomplished its purpose because reinforcement was established and Amanda's behaviour during the teaching sessions could be considered to have been brought under the control of her mother or the teacher.

Vocal Imitations as the Terminal Behaviour.

Motor imitation by Amanda was not the terminal behaviour which her mother set out to teach: three imitative speech sounds was the goal (see Appendix III). As the motor training continued, Amanda's mother vocalised (for example, "b" as in baby or ball) each time she reinforced Amanda. After two weeks of teaching in this way it was observed that Amanda also

---

* Videotape used: High Density J Standard Sony AV 34/20: Portapack.
** These figures are based on an average tally of two ten minute training sessions per day five days per week.

vocalised when she was not reinforced. Her mother then began to reinforce these vocalisations ("Good! Good Girl, Amanda") . . . usually followed by giving her a raisin or crisp or the lick of icecream, and slowly she thinned or dropped out the motor imitation. By the sixth week (sixtieth training session*) (see Fig. 7.4) Amanda was capable of two correct and sequential vocal imitations. By the ninth week (ninetieth training session*) Amanda had achieved a criterion of three correct sequential imitations and this result was confirmed in the tenth week, so that it could justifiably be concluded that criterion on this expressive language task had been achieved (see Fig. 7.4).

Reinforcement and Vocal Imitation

By the end of the third week (thirtieth training session) Amanda's mother was able to drop out the motor imitation and obtain vocalisation by giving Amanda raisins, or, on occasions, icecream, and much praise as positive reinforcers. Although vocalisations had been shaped with these procedures, it was still necessary in the weeks that followed (weeks 4 to 10, see Fig. 7.4) to continue to teach Amanda to directly imitate speech sounds. This was accomplished by continually using reinforcement to shift Amanda's spontaneous utterances to imitations of her mother's vocal model. A vocal model (phoneme) was presented by Amanda's mother and Amanda's imitation of the phoneme was followed by giving Amanda a raisin and plenty of praise. This procedure was also used in the independent testing at the end of each week. When Amanda's emission of three correctly imitated phonemes (/a/ as in *ma* or *father*, /i/ /ee/ as in *me* or *feet*, /b/ as in *big* or *boat*) had been brought under echoic control (in the tenth week, one hundredth training session*) then word teaching began in expressive language exercises III and IV (see Appendix II and Appendix III).

Conclusion

It is one thing to teach a child specific responses and utterances through means of a controlling teaching technique and another to get the child to generalise and retain what has apparently been learned. The gains made by Amanda during the specific target teaching programme O_2 to O_5 need to be seen alongside her measured receptive and expressive language scores over the thirty three months of the programme O_1 to O_6. Amanda's Columbia Mental Maturity Scale Score (Burgmeister et al., 1972) placed her in the first percentile at the start of the programme at O_1 and this did not change even after repeated testing (O_1 to O_6 inclusive). This assessment would appear to be confirmed by Amanda's performance on the Reynell Language Test over this period. Table 7.5 illustrates Amanda's receptive and expressive language age scores in months throughout the duration of the programme.

The conclusions to be drawn from these data and from Amanda's behaviour at the end of the programme are as follows:

(i) There is evidence during the nine months of the treatment programme O_2 to O_5 that Amanda's expressive language skills improved as shown by her achieving criterion levels in Expressive Language Tasks II and III, and also by the improved expressive language scores of five to thirteen months from O_2 to O_4. However, despite this evidence, it was clear that Amanda's flow of speech was still severely hampered, and in Expressive Language Task II (naming of body parts) Amanda's articulation was never clear and even this required an enormous effort and concentration. Sounds and words were producing very slowly. Speaking for Amanda required such an effort that every attempt was made to communicate by gesture. This extreme effort meant that for speaking to be maintained, it always had to be effectively reinforced. In the absence of effectively shaping and reinforcing Amanda's speech then she resorted to the use of gesture, and it is felt that this is demonstrated by the decline in her expressive language scores from thirteen months to seven months — O_4 to O_5 and O_6.

(ii) The achievement of criterion levels in Receptive Language Tasks IV, XIV, XV, XVI and XVII, demonstrated that Amanda could achieve criterion in a structured task that was

---

* These figures are based on an average tally of two ten minute training sessions per day five days per week.

TABLE 7.5

Amanda's Reynell Developmental
Language Age Scores in Months.

	0_1	0_2	0_3	0_4	0_5	0_6
Receptive Language Age	20	23	22	24	23	27
Expressive Language Age	05*	05	13	13	07	07
Chronological Age	49	61	64	67	70	82

* 0_5 months was the language recorded wherever a child failed to reach
the minimum language age score on the Reynell Language Test (Reynell
1969b) of 6 months.

rehearsed and effectively reinforced. However, this did not generalise to the Reynell Language Test as no improvement in the comprehension receptive language scores took place over the period of testing 0_2 to 0_5 (see Fig. 3.1). The four months' gain score (twenty-three months to twenty-seven months) from 0_5 to 0_6 needs to take into account that Amanda was one year older. It may be, therefore, that with increasing motivation and maturity, her receptive language ability will continue to slowly improve, and that whilst specific responses can be taught, there is little evidence that, to date, they generalise to other situations.

CASE STUDY III AND IV

Teaching Prepositional Requests

Subjects

Case Study III — Mary is a four years five months old Down's syndrome girl, the third of four children. She lived at home and attended a local Special School. She was diagnosed as severely retarded with a Stanford Binet (Form LM) score assessed at 35. Her Reynell Receptive Language Age was assessed at 28 months and Expressive Language Age at 15 months (Reynell, 1969b). She had good eye contact and was quite capable of initiating social interaction with others. She used toys most appropriately.

Case Study IV — Justin is a nine year old boy residing at home. He was the seventh of eight children in the family. His diagnosis was moderately to severely retarded (of no known organic origin) and he was also described as "reluctant and somewhat withdrawn". Justin had some communicable speech but rarely responded to verbal requests unless they were accompanied by much gesture. However, he could follow simple instructions, he could identify "most common objects" but did not respond correctly to prepositional requests. His Stanford Binet (Form LM) IQ score at 0_1 was assessed at 43. His Reynell Receptive Language Age at 0_2 was assessed at 31 months and his Reynell Expressive Language Age at 0_2 was 22 months (Reynell, 1969b).

Teaching Procedure

Mary and her parents and Justin and his mother had been involved in the preparatory stage I of the language training programme. Mary had been in a developmental speech therapy Group C for the first six months of this programme and Justin had been in the social work/supportive counselling Group B (see above Ch. 3). It was after this time that both Mary and Justin joined the target teaching language group (see above Ch. 3 p. 58 and Ch. 4 Fig. 4.2) and came to undertake the preposition language tasks.

Each week the parents attended group training sessions in the use of behaviourally oriented target teaching (see Ch. 3, p. 58) as well as one individual clinic teaching session per week. Part of the contract for the target teaching group at this stage was that the parents undertake a **minimum** of two ten minute teaching sessions per day, at least five days per week, and that they bring their recording sheets to the group training sessions and submit the results to the experimenter and to other members of the parent group for discussion. Criterion probes were carried out each week on the task by independent teachers who were not involved in the parent training programme in either the group or individual sessions. The group training took place with other families whose children were on similar tasks. Adjacent to the group training room were 2m x 2m clinic teaching rooms with one way screens. It was in these rooms that parents observed the teacher working with the child and themselves undertook supervised teaching of the relevant prepositional tasks.

Prepositional Language Tasks

After discussion with parents, five requests, using everyday items, were devised for each locational prepositional category (see Table 7.6). This meant that there were fifteen separate request items, five for each category, for both teaching and probe sessions. Objects that had appeared in previous language tasks were used for the direct object. Different objects were used for the object of the preposition (Table 7.6).

TABLE 7.6

Location Prepositions for Case Studies III and IV

Preposition for Teaching Requests	Preposition Probe Requests
"in the" requests	**"in the" requests**
Put the ball **in** the bucket.	Put the block **in** the box.
Put the ball **in** the cupboard.	Put the car **in** the garage.
Put the doll **in** the box.	Put the cup **in** the cupboard.
Put the keys **in** the cupboard.	Put the keys **in** the box.
Put the sock **in** the shoe.	Put the spoon **in** the cup.
"on the" requests	**"on the" requests**
Put the book **on** the table.	Put the ball **on** the bed.
Put the car **on** the box.	Put the cup **on** the saucer.
Put the doll **on** the bed.	Put the cushion **on** the chair.
Put the sock **on** the chair.	Put the keys **on** the table.
Put the spoon **on** the plate.	Put the shoe **on** the floor.
"under the" requests	**"under the" requests**
Put the ball **under** the hat.	Put the book **under** the drum.
Put the block **under** the box.	Put the doll **under** the bucket.
Put the car **under** the bucket.	Put the keys **under** the cup.
Put the shoe **under** the chair.	Put the shoe **under** the table.
Put the stool **under** the table.	Put the sock **under** the hat.

Parents requested that the tasks had to be both meaningful and capable of being relevant to everyday family life. As often as possible each object was used for each category of request. Therefore, each child had to attend to the prepositional cues in order to respond correctly. During any one probe session the probe requests were randomly presented. To make a request (e.g. "put the spoon in the cup") the tester in the probe sessions placed the object (the spoon) and the object of the preposition (in this case the cup) on the table in front of the child. Then the tester waited

173

until the child was quiet and looking at him before verbally making the request. This procedure was also part of the parent group and individual training, and was carried out in the child's home during teaching sessions. Individual clinic teaching sessions were videotaped* as were a random selection of parent teaching sessions in the home. In both of these teaching sessions, the request to be taught was presented to the child, and if s/he reponded correctly s/he was praised. It should be emphasised here that the use of food (chips, sweets or icecream) as a reinforcer was discussed with the parents and they rejected this, preferring to use praise (see Ch. 3, p. 56). If, in these teaching sessions in the clinic or at home, the child made no response to the request within ten seconds of its presentation, then the teacher or the parent prompted him by physically guiding him through the response (Mittler, 1975; Wright, Clayton and Edgar, 1970), and immediately delivered praise. An incorrect response produced "No" and a headshake from the parent, followed by a minimum ten second period when the teacher or mother remained silent. Then the request was presented again, and the child prompted for the correct response. As soon as the correct response (e.g. spoon **in** the cup) had been produced then praise followed immediately. Physical prompts were faded out over a number of teaching sessions by gradually reducing the physical dimensions of the prompts until the subjects, Mary or Justin, were responding correctly to the verbal requests without assistance. The teaching procedure continued until either child reached a criterion of five correct responses without prompting (Fig. 7.6). The session was then terminated. If criterion was not reached in a teaching session either in the clinic room or at home then teaching of the same task was continued in the next session. As soon as Mary or Justin had achieved criterion on one set of prepositional requests, as established in the weekly probe sessions, then the **next** prepositional request (e.g. "on the" request) was taught. As soon as the criterion had been achieved on this prepositional request then discrimination training between the "in the" and the "on the" requests began.

Discrimination teaching consisted of concurrent teaching on one request (e.g. "put the book on the table"), from another request (e.g. "put the ball under the hat", or "put the ball in the bucket"). In initial discrimination teaching different pairs of objects were used for each request. However, once criterion had been achieved on each request separately, using the same object (e.g. "put the ball in the bucket", or "put the ball on the chair", or "put the ball under the hat"), then any combination of prepositional requests was presented randomly. Requests in probe sessions were also presented in random order, and criterion performance was reached when the subject responded correctly to any combination of six prepositional requests. When criterion was reached, the teaching sessions on these preposition receptive language tasks were terminated and selection and teaching on the next language task in the language manual began.

Scoring of responses

A correct response to an "in the" request was recorded by the mother at home and the tester in the weekly probe sessions when the subject placed the direct object (e.g. sock — in the request "put the sock in the shoe"), in the object of the preposition — in this case, the shoe. In daily home teaching this request was presented five times and correct responses were recorded (see Figures 7.6 and 7.7). Parents had to present the daily data recording chart each week to the experimenter at the weekly group training sessions. Similar recording procedures were used for the "on the" requests. For the "under the" requests a correct response was recorded if, when required, the subject lifted the object of the preposition and placed the direct object under it and then removed his hands from both objects (e.g. lifting the cup and putting the keys directly **under** the upturned cup or placing a stool adjacent to a table **under** the table). Toys were used in the clinic training sessions but parents were encouraged to relate the tasks to real objects wherever possible.

Reliability was achieved by checking the child's responses in the weekly probe sessions, by getting the parents to bring the daily data recording chart to weekly group sessions, and also by randomly videotaping home based teaching sessions.

* Videotapes used: High Density J Standard Sony AV 34/20: Portapack.

174

Separating the requests

There was clear evidence that the children had much difficulty in discriminating between untaught "in the", "on the" and "under the" requests. This occurs even though these are definite spatial prepositions in which actions or events that may occur can be used to establish comprehension. Therefore, to begin with, these requests were taught separately. There were five situations to be taught and probed. These were: (i) "in the" requests alone; (ii) "on the" requests alone; (iii) "in the" and "on the" requests together; (iv) "under the" requests separately, and (v) "in the" "on the" and "under the" requests together. Probing continued in alternation with clinic and home based teaching until the child correctly responded to all of the "in the", "on the" and "under the" requests. When the child responded correctly to each request separately then discrimination training was initiated and weekly probes then took place to assess whether generalisation had occurred. This probing for generalisation alternated with training until the child (Mary or Justin) correctly responded to all the prepositional requests (see Table 7.6), no matter what objects were used. Discrimination teaching in the clinic and at home continued until the child responded to all of the prepositional requests in the probe sessions for at least two consecutive probe sessions. More than two probe sessions for this language task took place if the parent, in conjunction with the clinic teachers, felt that more teaching of these skills was necessary, despite the fact that criterion had been achieved in the daily home teaching and in the previous probe session.

Prepositional Requests Results

CASE STUDY III — Mary's results

The graphs of Figure 7.6 show Mary's performance on the daily teaching at home. The pre-test sessions, when Mary's language profile was constructed, demonstrated that she did not respond appropriately to any of the probe requests as outlined in Table 7.6. In the home based teaching sessions her mother recorded that she made no errors on the "in the" requests after the ninth teaching session (45 presentations of this stimulus command "put the ball in the bucket" etc). This was verified in the probe sessions at the end of the first week and confirmed at the end of the second week. Mary achieved criterion for the "on the" requests after one individual clinic teaching session and seven home teaching sessions (this involved a minimum of 35 presentations of the stimulus command "put the car on the box", etc.).

The third task was a discrimination training condition in which the "in the" and "on the" requests were concurrently taught between each probe session. Mary's performance on the "in the" training requests remained nearly as errorless, but for the "on the" requests her performance fluctuated, and it is this fluctuation that was responsible for the error rate in the first five home teaching sessions (see Figure 7.6). However, after a minimum* of 13 teaching sessions Mary achieved criterion (five out of five) by successfully discriminating between the "in the" and "on the" requests when presented randomly, and this was confirmed in the probe sessions at the end of the third week.

Criterion for the "under the" requests was achieved after a minimum* of 11 home teaching sessions (see Figure 7.6). This involved a minimum of 55 presentations of the stimulus command "put the block under the box", etc.

Situation (v) was designed to teach discrimination among all three requests. Mary's parents were determined to complete the task successfully. The parents understood that probe sessions would again be based on a random presentation of six requests, including any combination of each of the three categories. It should be stressed that before a teaching session (either individual, clinic, or at home) in which a new request was to be introduced, Mary was rehearsed on pointing to the objects named. The errors made on the forty-fifth, forty-sixth and forty-seventh teaching sessions (see Figure 7.6) were due to confusion among the prepositional requests, and Mary's failure to achieve any correct responses in the fifty-second and fifty-third teaching sessions (see

---

*   These figures are based on the two ten minute **recorded** teaching sessions per day for a minimum of five days per week. Other home teaching did take place but this was not recorded.

FIGURE 7.6

Sessional graphical record of Mary's
correct responses to location preposi tonal
responses *

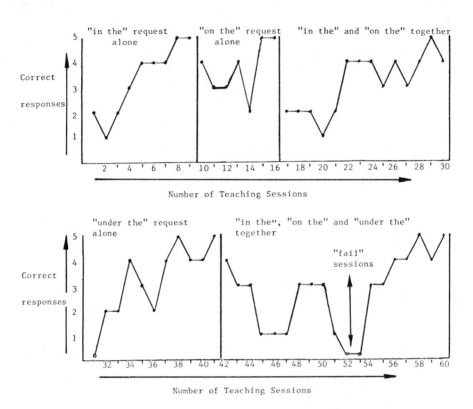

Number of Teaching Sessions

Number of Teaching Sessions

* The termination of a task and the onset of the next task
means that criterion has been achieved in both home teaching
and probe sessions.

Figure 7.6) was ascribed by Mary's mother to Mary being unwell and "therefore, somewhat indifferent" on those particular teaching sessions. Criterion performance was attained on the fifty-eighth home teaching session and again on the sixtieth session (see Figure 7.6). This result was confirmed in the probe session at the end of the sixth week. Therefore, after six individual clinic teaching sessions, six probe sessions, and a minimum* of 60 home based teaching sessions, Mary was able to discriminate between distinct locational prepositional requests and could generalise these no matter what known objects were involved.

* These figures are based on the two ten minute **recorded** teaching sessions per day for a minimum of five days per week. Other home teaching did take place but this was not recorded.

CASE STUDY IV — Justin's results.

The graphs of Figure 7.7 show Justin's performance on the daily teaching at his home. The baseline sessions at 0_2 when Justin's language profile was assessed, demonstrated that he did not respond appropriately to any of the probe requests on the location preposition tasks. In the teaching sessions (see Figure 7.7) Justin achieved criterion for the "in the" requests on the thirteenth home teaching session (a minimum of 60 presentations of the stimulus command "put the sock in the shoe" etc.), and this performance was repeated in the fourteenth recorded home teaching session, and verified in the probe sessions at the end of the second week.

The second prepositional request, the "on the" request, proved as difficult at the start as the "in the" request. After 16 sessions Justin had failed to achieve criterion (five out of five) on either the teaching sessions or the probe sessions. At this point the recording of teaching on this task was

FIGURE 7.7

Sessional graphical record of Justin's
correct responses to location prepositional
requests *

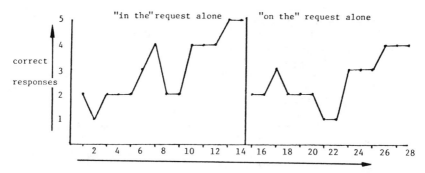

Number of Teaching Sessions

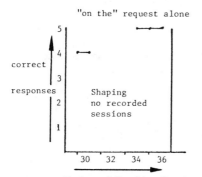

Number of Teaching Sessions

* The termination of a task and the onset of the next
task means that criterion has been achieved in both
home teaching and probe sessions.

discontinued while Justin's mother, helped by the clinic teacher, shaped Justin's behaviour by physically guiding his responses. For example, his mother took Justin's hand and placed it on the spoon and then physically placed the spoon on the plate, or, alternatively, carried out the same shaping procedure with the car and the box. Each time this shaping procedure took place, Justin's mother emphasised the prepositional cue **"on the"**. After three intervening shaping sessions (see Figure 7.7) Justin achieved criterion (five out of five) and this was repeated in the two following teaching sessions. Justin also responded correctly in the probe sessions at the end of the fourth week.

Justin did not receive discrimination training for the "in the" and "on the" requests together. Justin was slow to respond in both the teaching and probe sessions, frequently attending to the object cues. After discussion, his mother indicated that she preferred to undertake teaching of "an easier task" despite the fact that Justin achieved criterion for the "on the" requests immediately after the shaping sessions and the additional stress on emphasising the prepositional cues. Therefore, Justin shifted to receptive language task XII (see Appendix II) "pairing related objects". This task was considered somewhat easier than the discrimination skill necessary for criterion to be achieved on all the prepositional requests.

Discussion of Results: The Problems of Generalisation

The teaching for both these children demonstrates that severely intellectually handicapped children can be taught by their parents to follow prepositional instructions through the use of modelling, shaping, prompting, and reinforcement procedures. In addition, the results show that as the children learned to respond to prepositional requests of one category, their responses to untrained requests of those categories became increasingly correct. Furthermore, in the subject Mary's case, her results showed an ability to discriminate between prepositional categories on untrained requests. These results replicate the receptive language research of Baer and Guess (1971) and Frisch and Schumaker (1974).

These teaching sessions were carried out in the home and there are some problems to be considered, particularly in the teaching of discriminations. In these cases it was necessary to teach and obtain generalisation in each category separately before teaching a discrimination between categories and obtaining generalisation of that discrimination. This sequence of conditions applied in Mary's case, even though she achieved criterion on all five tasks. It was felt that Justin's criterion responses on the thirty-fourth, thirty-fifth, and thirty-sixth teaching sessions, and in the probe session at the end of the fourth week, were indicative that he could have progressed to the discrimination tasks (iii) and (v). However, by this stage, his mother had decided that these discrimination tasks would have resulted in "some more disruption at home", especially if Justin had failed in the tasks. This problem of parents' unwillingness to persist with home teaching when they don't perceive that they are having much success has to be both accepted and tackled. At this stage, the pressures of domestic routines for Justin's mother, plus the fact that she perceived him to have had much difficulty with the first two categories, resulted in his not continuing with training on the discrimination tasks. It remains to be determined whether Justin could have achieved criterion on these tasks. Certainly, a family counselling programme, which stressed the importance of the auditory prepositional cues, and which set out to convince the family that Justin was capable of learning to make discriminations, would have helped at this stage. The fact is that he had learned to generalise to untrained requests of each category separately. This was considered a prerequisite for making the discrimination between categories of prepositional requests together, even though in both the individual clinic teaching and the home teaching, he had given much attention to the visual object cues rather than the auditory prepositional cues. Nevertheless, in the probe sessions, when he was asked to respond to requests when the previously learned object cues were not available, he was able to make that discrimination.

It does appear that by achieving criterion on the probe requests in the first two categories, both Mary and Justin had achieved generalisation without the use of any visual cue. However, visual cues, such as familiar objects, had been integral in commencing and sustaining the home based teaching. This would seem to support Sailor and Taman's point of view that the use of extraneous cues might help children to learn discriminations (Sailor and Taman, 1972). This was certainly the case in the first stages of teaching prepositional usage in the home to both children.

This teaching programme has been designed for use by parents in their homes. Certainly, the individual clinic teaching took place in a laboratory setting. Certainly, the parents were encouraged to teach in a setting in which needed objects were within easy reach and in which there were as few extraneous distractions as possible. However, it was felt that by training parents to teach their children in their homes, this was a very close approximation to the natural environment. Common household objects were used in the teaching sessions. In both the teaching and the probe sessions the child was close to the objects. The next stage of teaching of the prepositional requests is to increase the distance between the child and the named objects so that the child is still able to respond to the auditory cue while also having to locate the object. In addition, different prepositions, such as "next to" (e.g. in an instruction "put your shoes **next to** Sally's") or "for" (e.g. in a request "please get my shoes **for** me") could be taught. However, there may be a definite limit to specific teaching of the types of prepositions and situations in which they can be used. Fries (1952) has reported that there are 250 possible meanings for the nine prepositions (of, in, to, for, at, on, from, with, by), which comprise 90 per cent of the prepositions in written materials. There are few patterns which indicate the appropriate use of prepositions, and to introduce many others might well cause much confusion.

It is possible to enlarge an intellectually handicapped child's receptive language repertoire by teaching prepositions, particularly those which denote spatial aspects. Yet the success of such a teaching programme will depend on vital parent variables, such as teaching skill and persistence. The older the child, the more likely it is that s/he will be less open to developing a receptive language repertoire. Furthermore, when confusion and complexity appear with the introduction of additional prepositions, then the child's abstraction and generalisation problems may become more acute. As such, for any one child, there may be definite limits to the types of prepositions he can understand, no matter how skilled the teaching. Parents and teachers need to be aware of this so that teaching goals are realistic, and success for both child and parent is ensured, thus strengthening and supporting parents' persistence in carrying out the programme.

CASE STUDY V

(i) Identifying pictures for general descriptions.
(ii) Describing pictures by using noun phrases.

The subject, Gerald, is a ten year old Down's Syndrome boy*, the eighth and last born child of the family. His assessed mean Stanford Binet IQ score was forty-four[ø] and his performance on the Columbia Mental Maturity Scale (Burgmeister et al. 1972) at O_2 placed Gerald in the first percentile. Gerald was well able to **imitate** basic sounds in words or, indeed, whole words. His assessed language ages on the Reynell Developmental Language Scales (Reynell 1969b) at O_2 when his teaching programme began were: Reynell Receptive Language Age (RRLA) 50 months and Reynell Expressive Language Age (RELA) 31 months. This expressive language age score at O_2 was accepted although it did appear very low in comparison with what Gerald was able to achieve in both observed teaching situations and in subsequent testing situations. In fact, his mean expressive language age (RELA) for the six testing sessions O_1 to O_6 inclusive was 48.2 months. This is felt to be more representative of Gerald's overall expressive language ability, but his very low expressive language age at O_2 is included here because it does indicate the fluctuations in measured performance that could occur for Gerald or, indeed, for many other intellectually handicapped children in the programme.

---

*   Nine years old at the commencement of the programme at O_1, therefore ten years old at the beginning of the case study at O_2.

[ø]   Mean Stanford Binet IQ score reported here is the average of his IQ scores at O_2 and O_6 (see Fig. 3.1. Ch. 3).

Gerald's family situation was close and supporting. Older brothers and sisters occasionally attended the group teaching sessions and certainly practised specific language tasks at home. However, it was Gerald's mother who carried out the teaching at home on a regular basis and who was videotaped when teaching Gerald. Gerald's father also attended five of the group training sessions for Target Teaching Group A (see above Ch. 3) and he clearly provided consistent and enthusiastic support for the mother's teaching. Furthermore, there is clear evidence from school records that regular teaching at home had been an accepted part of family life since his birth. His mother was familiar with many of the language teaching skills developed in this programme. Certainly, Gerald displayed much motivation, a developed attention span and comprehensive verbal imitation skills. The extent to which Gerald's family rehearsed language tasks "at every available opportunity" may also account for his speed of response and effective memory.

Receptive Language Tasks mastered by Gerald during the period of teaching 0_2 to 0_5 (see above Fig. 3.1)

The receptive language tasks indicated below are those successfully completed by Gerald during the teaching period. These three tasks (R.L. XXIV, Counting task with various objects, two five object sets; R.L. XXV, Counting task with various objects, three five object sets and R.L. XXXII, Auditory/visual association exercise) were the only receptive language tasks that Gerald had failed to achieve criterion on when his baseline language profile was assessed at 0_2 (see Appendices II and V).

Receptive Language Task XXXIV

This language task explores Gerald's ability to respond to quite categorical names by correctly associating the stimulus command with a particular picture. The recorded teaching took

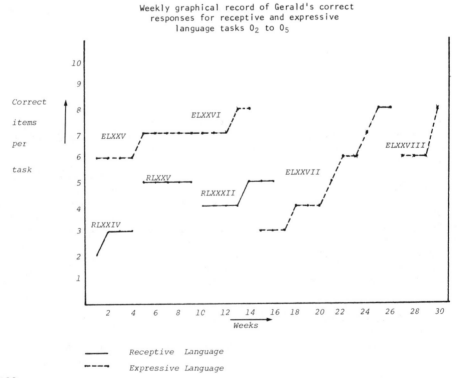

FIGURE 7.8

Weekly graphical record of Gerald's correct
responses for receptive and expressive
language tasks 0_2 to 0_5

180

place in the family dining room, or once a week in a small 3m by 2m room at Gerald's special school. The teaching procedure for Gerald was as follows:

(i) His mother placed two pictures on the table in front of him; for example, a picture of a house and a picture of a pencil.

(ii) His mother said "Point to . . . " or "Give me a picture of something that we live in!" Gerald was then expected to discriminate between the picture of the house and the picture of the pencil and give his mother the picture of the house. It needs to be stressed that the request "Give me a picture of something that we live in!" is quite distinct and more difficult than a command "Give me a picture of a house!"

(iii) As soon as Gerald could distinguish between the picture of the house and the picture of the pencil by giving his mother either picture within ten seconds of the requisite command ("Give me a picture of something that we live in!" or "Give me a picture of something that we draw with!"), then a third card with a picture of an aeroplane was added to the other two. The teaching procedure requesting Gerald to distinguish one card from another and then give it to his mother was carried out as before, with Gerald's mother randomly presenting the commands "Give me something that we draw with!", "Give me something that we fly in!" or "Give me something that we live in!" Gerald's mother prompted him whenever he showed uncertainty or had difficulty with the task. The prompts in the early stages involved gesture, or, when an error was made, actually placing Gerald's finger on the picture related to the command. His mother reinforced all correct responses with a quietly spoken, but definite, "Good boy, Gerald. That's right!" looking directly at him as she did so.

(iv) When criterion of being able to distinguish between any of three pictures (house, pencil, aeroplane) had been achieved a fourth picture (a picture of a knife and fork) with the related command "Give me a picture of something that we eat with" was added to the previous three pictures. As soon as Gerald had achieved criterion on this task then a fifth and final picture (picture of a car) with the related command "Give me something that we ride in!" was added to the other four. Criterion of this receptive language task was considered to have been achieved when Gerald could discriminate and select the appropriate card from among the four distractors in a picture choice situation.

Results

Fig. 7.8 illustrates that Gerald took seven weeks (weeks ten to sixteen inclusive) to achieve criterion on this task. Using the formula of a minimum of two ten minute teaching sessions five times a week, then Gerald achieved criterion on this task after a minimum of seventy teaching sessions. During the first four weeks of independent testing (weeks ten to thirteen) Gerald always managed to select four cards correctly. Observation of his teaching sessions revealed that he was often confused as to whether he should name the picture on the card (since his mother always stressed that he should be able to name the objects) or give his mother the card. However, Gerald's mother, in concentrating on teaching Gerald to imitate words (particularly nouns to begin with) and then to produce spoken responses at random, insisted that she had aided his comprehension. Certainly, Gerald's responses on many of the receptive language or comprehension tasks were both quicker (in response time) and superior (he achieved criterion with fewer teaching sessions) to those children who had difficulty in imitating the nouns or, indeed, could not say the same imitated words without an imitative stimulus. The fact that the stimulus command did not name the picture card directly, ("Give me a picture of something that we live in!" rather than "Give me a picture of a house!") certainly makes this comprehension task more difficult than if the picture were named directly. However, the fact that Gerald could say all the names of the objects on the cards (house, pencil, car, knife and fork, aeroplane or "plane") was a necessary referent for him in comprehending the less specific and more general commands.

Expressive Language Task XXVII — Noun Phrase and Description

Gerald achieved criterion of eight correct responses out of any ten different presentations (see Fig. 7.9) of the stimulus command "What is happening here?" or "Tell me what is happening here!", after twelve weeks of teaching, and a minimum of one hundred and twenty structured teaching sessions. This expressive language task is a development of previous expressive language tasks mastered by Gerald, for example, the ability to correctly name objects in specific relationship to room parts (E.L. XII, see Appendix II and Appendix III) or the correct use of three verbs with a specific object (E.L. XV, see Appendix II and Appendix III). Certainly, his mastery of Expressive Language Task XXV (E.L. XXV), sentence response to the question "What can you see?" (objects), (successfully completed in nine weeks and ninety teaching sessions) and Expressive Language Task XXVI (E.L. XXVI), sentence response to the question "What can you see?" (pictures), (successfully completed in five weeks and fifty teaching sessions) (see Appendix II and Expressive Language Tasks, Appendix III) under structured teaching conditions could be considered as suitable preparation for the more linguistically advanced expressive language task involving noun phrase and description (E.L. XXVIII).

Daily Teaching

The expressive language responses taught by Gerald's mother followed the presentation of particular pictures. The pictures were as follows:

Picture	Required Response
1. Man sitting on a bench.	Man on seat, or, A man sitting on a seat.
2. Boy crossing the road.	A boy crossing the road, or, Boy crossing road.
3. Car in a garage.	Car in garage.
4. Boy up a tree.	Boy in a tree, or, Boy up a tree.
5. Ducks on a pond.	Ducks on the pond, or, Duck on pond.
6. Girl with a dog.	A girl with a dog, or, Girl with dog.
7. Lamb in a field.	A lamb in a field, or, Lamb in field.
8. Airliner in flight.	Aeroplane in flight, or, Plane flying, or, Plane in air.

The aim of this exercise was to obtain a meaningful and understood noun phrase response from the child. The teaching procedure was as follows:
  (i) Gerald and his mother were seated at the dining room table. Gerald's mother had the stimulus cards.
 (ii) Gerald's mother presented the first card (the picture of the man on a bench) and then said "Gerald, tell me what is happening here!"
(iii) Gerald's mother prompted him by pointing first to the man and then to the bench, saying each word as she did so.
(iv) Gerald responded by saying "Man bench" and then, with prompting "Man on bench". The same teaching strategy was applied with picture card 2 (Boy crossing the road) and picture card 3 (Car in a garage). The telegraphic responses were noted but regarded as achieving criterion. Given a visual cue, Gerald was well able to first imitate and then produce a one word response in context.

Results
1. By the end of the first week, Gerald had achieved criterion on the first three picture cards: that is, he was able to correctly respond to the statements "What is happening here?" or "What is this?" when the picture cards were presented to him. The words clearly produced by Gerald were "Man", "on", "bench", "boy", "road", "in" and "car". He uttered the word "cross" (but not "crossing") when prompted, and in the independent testing, his approximation to "cross" or "crossing" was accepted. The definite article "the" was not produced, though observation revealed that Gerald could imitate the word. It should be noted that, apart from the **minimum** two ten minute teaching sessions per day, five days a week, Gerald's family admitted to "hours of initial training" until Gerald could spontaneously identify and name the objects on the cards.
2. Over a period of a **minimum** of thirty teaching sessions during the first three weeks, Gerald had achieved a fluency on these cards with a speed of response often inside two seconds, and generally an acceptable response within five seconds. The fourth card (Boy up a tree) had been introduced in the second week, but after discussion with Gerald's mother, he had not

been tested on this card until the fourth week, so as to minimise any failure experiences which "so reduce Gerald's motivation".

3. Many of the words in the noun phrase description of cards 4, 5, 6 and 7, were already a part of Gerald's repertoire, ("Boy", "tree", "duck", "on", "up", "in", "girl", "dog", "lamb") and had been both rehearsed in previous language tasks and used in the family in what can best be described as imitative learning situations by Gerald, based on effective modelling by his family and aided by distinct verbal and visual cues. By the sixth week (sixtieth teaching session) Gerald had achieved criterion on picture cards 1 to 6 and could produce the following utterances (see also Fig. 7.8), "Man on bench", "Boy cross . . . road", "Car in garage" (pronounced "grage!"), "Boy in tree", "Duck on pond", "Girl with dog". Furthermore, these utterances did transfer to the classroom situation where immediate social reinforcement followed correct noun phrase utterances.

4. By the end of the tenth week (week twenty-four, see Fig. 7.8) Gerald's mother had taught Gerald the word "field" by modelling imitation, careful and immediate social reinforcement with each successive approximation to the word "field" and controlled verbal prompting. The independent testing at week twenty-four demonstrated that Gerald could produce the seven noun phrase utterances when the stimulus picture cards were randomly presented to him. Despite the carefully structured testing situation with which Gerald was familiar, these responses did provide evidence of a developing memory span and a definite ability to produce two and three word sentences.

FIGURE 7.9

Sessional graphical record of Gerald's correct responses
for Expressive Language Task XXVII (the accepted response
appears beneath each graph - words or word endings in parentheses
were taught but appear only intermittently in Gerald's responses)

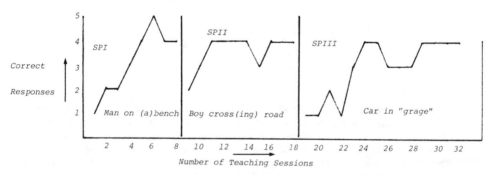

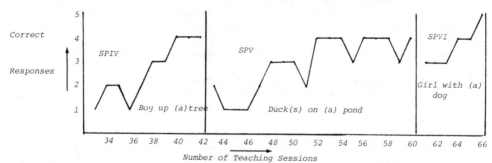

SP _____ Stimulus Picture

183

FIGURE 7.9 (continued)

Sessional graphical record of Gerald's correct responses
for Expressive Language Task XXVII (the accepted response
appears beneath each graph - words or word endings in parentheses
were taught but appear only intermittently in Gerald's responses)

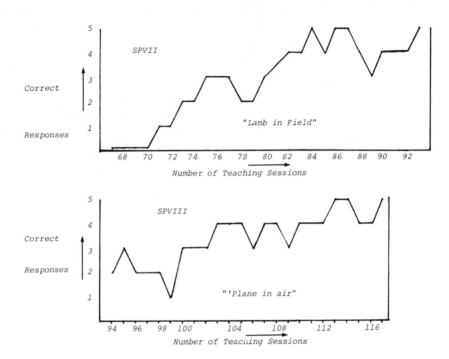

5. During the eleventh and twelfth week of teaching on this task (weeks twenty-five and twenty-six) Gerald was able to utter the words "plane", "in" and "air". At both the teaching and independent testing sessions he imitated a 'plane in flight with his hands and his response to the picture of an airline in flight depended on the contextual play, and the response was laboured. However, the fact that the independent tester provided the appropriate visual cues was regarded as acceptable because no child should be expected to produce vocabulary in isolation. Furthermore, there was evidence from previous noun and noun phrase utterances, that the quality of Gerald's utterances would improve greatly with time. Certainly, if attention was paid to always carefully structuring the situation, then motivation would be maintained and a generalisation effect of the utterances learned could be anticipated.

Relationship between Gerald's Receptive and Expressive Language

Examination of Gerald's responses during the ninth month of teaching reveals the following relationship between his receptive language (auditory comprehension) and expressive language (productive speech):

1. that in common with normative studies of language development such as the research studies carried out by Fraser, Bellugi and Brown (1963) and Shipley, Smith and Gleitman (1969) and with theoretical positions taken up by Myklebust (1957) and Chomsky (1967), there is clear evidence that Gerald's receptive or comprehension ability **preceded** the development

of productive speech. For example, upon entry into the programme, Gerald already possessed high skills in pointing to named objects, selecting numbers of different objects and, as the programme progressed, he was able to respond correctly to singular or plural labelled commands and to more abstract commands, as in the case of Receptive Language Exercise XXXII above. At the time of being able to respond correctly to these tasks Gerald could not say the words involved;

2. that during the period of structured reinforced teaching, Gerald was taught labelling skills to an errorless criterion without this necessarily achieving generalisation. Furthermore, there is evidence from both his home and school situation, that these words were often used out of context or in a meaningless fashion, so much so, that there was evidence here that Gerald did not comprehend just what he was saying. This might be considered, therefore, to support Chapman and Miller's position that production actually precedes comprehension (Chapman and Miller, 1973);

3. that there is no specific evidence that teaching language skills in one repertoire (either receptive language or expressive language) would facilitate acquisition in the other repertoire. This may provide evidence that comprehension and production of speech are functionally independent. However, when the language tasks in receptive and expressive language were similar, if not identical, then training in one modality could be demonstrated to aid the development of skills in the other repertoire. For example, verbal training on Expressive Language Task VI, Naming concealed objects (see Appendix II and Appendix III) could be demonstrated to have enhanced Gerald's (or any other child's) receptive discrimination ability. Similarly, training on receptive language skills, such as searching for and identifying named concealed objects, Receptive Language Task IX (see Appendix II and Appendix III), can be demonstrated to have enhanced the similar Expressive Language Task VI, Naming concealed objects (see Appendix II and Appendix III).

The main conclusion that can be drawn from this study is that for Down's Syndrome children, a variety of relationships exist between receptive and expressive language. Some conditions under which a functional relationship can exist have been indicated and some other conditions, demonstrating independence of the modalities, have been shown. In Gerald's case, some generalisation between the two modalities, receptive and expressive language, can occur, but there is no evidence that it is automatic even in a teaching programme where every effort has been made in the selection and sequencing of tasks to emphasise the functional similarity of both modalities.

The Distinctiveness of Gerald's family's teaching and assessment

An important aspect of Gerald's mother's teaching was the close relationship between the family's description of his language ability during Stage I (see Chapter 3 above and Appendix V) and Gerald's performance on the criterion language tasks at 0_2. Gerald's parents had over the years proved to be reliable recorders of his behaviour. This is important in this case study (and, indeed, in many others) because when Gerald's language behaviour proceeded from its different baseline on any specified language task, then the changes described and recorded by his parents did accurately reflect Gerald's stage of language development. This reliability proved to be a skill which could be passed on to other parents, particularly to younger parents. For example, Gerald's parents accepted his limitations and were accurate and realistic in their assessment of his ability. They often expressed the point of view that they did not have the option of being "unreliable" in reporting Gerald's developing language skills. This family, particularly the mother, has demonstrated that thoroughly reliable measurement of Gerald's language skills could take place in the home setting.

This continual teaching and reliable recording in the home allowed observers to make decisions as to just what was responsible for a corresponding behavioural change. Clearly, in Gerald's case, his parents could demonstrate that their daily structured teaching was largely responsible for the occurrence of particular language skills. As such, his parents had achieved a degree of analysis of Gerald's language behaviour because they could exercise control over it. This may appear an arrogant claim in Gerald's parents' case. However, their measuring was highly reliable and they had taught, assessed and examined Gerald's behaviour for many months and years until in **their** eyes, the stability of the acquired language skills had been achieved. They had measured Gerald's developing language skills during the period of applying structured teaching and reinforcement procedures O_2 to O_5 (see Fig. 3.1). They had demonstrated the effectiveness of structured teaching and reinforcement procedures for producing change in Gerald's language skills, whether in receptive or expressive modality. They had always then been prepared to see if the language skills acquired under the structured teaching situation did generalise in the family's daily domestic life. If the acquired language skills were not maintained, then the systematic structured teaching was begun again or stepped up, since for Gerald's parents, the achievement of a language skill was considered to be most important. Repeated reversals of the behaviour were not tried because this would be contrary to the family's life style: the family were concerned to maintain the language skills acquired. Gerald's mother's consistent application of structured teaching and reinforcement procedures had produced what was for them valuable behaviour — this valuable behaviour meant that, for his family, Gerald became an even more acceptable member. For example, his acquired language skills, as described above, regularly met with extra experimental reinforcement in the family's social setting. Therefore, for Gerald, these receptive and expressive language skills, once established in structured teaching, were no longer dependent on the experimental techniques which created them.

Generality of Gerald's Language Skills

There is a close correspondence between the criterion assessment of Gerald's language skills at O_2, Gerald's family's report of his langue ability during Stage I (O_1 to O_2) and his Reynell Receptive and Expressive Language scores O_1 to O_6 inclusive. His language skills certainly proved durable in the "settings that he knows", in particular, his home and his school. Moreover, the improvement in his receptive and expressive language skills, taught in a structured setting, proved to have generality in that it endured in the year (Stage III, see Fig. 3.1) that followed the structured teaching. However, both Gerald's mother and his teachers reported that in non-familiar situations he was "withdrawn . . . and as such, poorly motivated" and could not produce his evident language skills in these "threatening" situations. Generality in Gerald's language behaviour was not, therefore, automatically accomplished in unfamiliar settings. It should not, however, be assumed in this case (or, indeed, in many others) that the structured teaching and language skills so acquired had failed when generalisation did not take place in a widespread form. In Gerald's case, the structured teaching procedure which had been so effective in developing his language skills in the home setting, could perhaps be repeated in other settings, and thus accomplish the generalisation sought. Evidence from this language intervention programme suggests the wisdom of planning for generalisation in the long term.

Case Studies: Some General Conclusions

The five case studies selected cover a wide range of language skills teaching. They demonstrate many of the problems involved for parents in continually teaching their children language skills and in assessing the outcomes. From the point of view of parents' teaching and from the children's developing language skills, the following general conclusions are made:

(i) that a high degree of structure in teaching, allied to effective reinforcement procedures, can be used in the home;

(ii) that the effectiveness of this teaching depends both on the close attention that the parents are able to give to pre-planning and also on the regularity of teaching;

(iii) that the particular language skills being taught have, as near as possible, to synchronise with the children's level of maturation, otherwise the language skill will disappear when the structured teaching and reinforcement procedures are not maintained.

(iv) that success in the form of small sequential steps that the child can just attain and then maintain need to be planned for both the parents and their children (see case study II above);

(v) that parental motivation in maintaining such an involved continual structured teaching programme depends not only on the child's developing language skills, but on the understanding and regular contact with teachers, speech therapists and other professional workers in the field;

(vi) that regular contact with professional workers is vital because teaching programmes such as those described above (with the many, many sessions involved before a skill is acquired), can impose **great stress** in families, in particular, because the teaching programmes need to be continual and long term (see case study IV above);

(vii) that the earlier in the child's life that parents are able to begin structured teaching, the more likely they are to maximise the language skill development of their children (see the case studies I and V above);

(viii) that in the case of the more handicapped children, the goal of a language teaching programme involves teaching simple communication skills (see case study II) for which, in the child's lifetime, the level of sophistication is quite limited;

(ix) that the language and communication skills of imitation, comprehension and speech production can be taught separately and, as such, show little relationship or interdependence. Yet it can also be demonstrated that imitation aids comprehension, that imitation aids the development of speech production, and that comprehension can occur without speech production or, in turn, is a necessary prerequisite of speech production;

(x) that the generalisation of language and communication skills to many different situations is what parents so desire, but that this is most unlikely to occur without pre-planning (see case study III above). This pre-planning involves a much greater understanding by the wider community of the careful structure, longer response time and effective reinforcement needed for the intellectually handicapped child to adequately communicate in an unfamiliar environment.

PART THREE

CONCLUSION

Chapter Eight

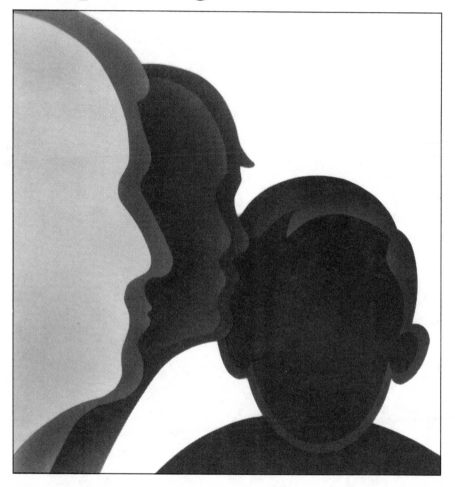

Conclusions and Recommendations
for Further Research

Some Answers to the Problems of this Study

Parents who participated had the opportunity to be involved in every stage of this research. They did participate in the planning of the research (see Ch. 3, p. 53), they could and did observe the language testing and had access to their children's results and their children's record files. The latter was an innovation. Parents' ideas were included in the language manual (see above Ch. 3, p. 57 and Appendix III). However, the need to produce the manual quickly at the end of Stage I (see Fig. 3.1, p. 54 and p. 57) meant that not as much careful consultation with parents took place as would have been desirable. Therefore the language manual was not as comprehensive as it might have been.

There was some technical language in the language manual that parents found of little value, for example, reference to auditory and visual modalities, or the particular references to articulation skills. There were no illustrations to help parents to understand particular teaching techniques. In fact the lack of illustrations was a major criticism revealed in the survey of parents' attitudes to the programme by Kimber and Porritt (1976).

The language manual assumed no verbal skills of the child at entry and terminated in the expressive language tasks at a level of simple sentence complexity. If a child's language problem was very specific for example, shifting from recognisable sounds to words, or developing particular comprehension strategies, or shifting from single words to two word open pivot utterances then the language manual was found to be too general and additional teaching materials had to be produced (see for example case studies III and IV in Ch. 7, p. 172). As such, parents could not identify with the written language programme which, because of its general nature did not necessarily help them with specific problems (see for example case study II, Ch. 7, p. 166).

It is well known that the ways in which reality is perceived are selective. Therefore whether or not the teaching programmes which took place during Stage II (see Ch. 3, pp. 57-61) were *realistic* depended on both parents' and professionals points of view. Parents' reasons for dislike of behaviour modification are identified in Ch. 2 (p. 30). The detailed teaching and perseverance that was required is apparent in the case studies presented in Chapter 7. The fact that this detailed teaching and perseverance was often an unrealistic expectation for many parents was indicated by the responses of parents to the PAAT survey (see Chapter 6). Certainly the parents who had a low score on the PAAT found the demands of daily teaching often to be unattainable and as such, unrealistic.

Heifetz (1977) described his instructional manuals as a self-contained resource. Maybe there is little correspondence between Heifetz's manuals and that used in this programme (see Appendix III). However both Heifetz's manuals and the one used here aim to teach similar skills, particularly those related to language development. However, for parents in the Language Programme only (Group D see Ch. 3, p. 61), the mere provision of a structured language manual without back-up professional support proved to be quite inadequate (see for example, Ch. 5, p. 113). As such, it would appear to be unrealistic to expect parents to persevere with teaching their intellectually handicapped children on a daily basis just because a comprehensive training package was provided.

This parent training intervention programme was sufficiently well funded so that the ratio of professionals (teachers, speech therapists, occupational therapists, counsellors) to parents was higher than is encountered in everyday service provision in departments of Health, Education and Welfare in the A.C.T. and surrounding districts. As such, the research represented a higher cost input than is normally provided. Whether or not it was a high cost programme, depends on parent and child benefit, in relation to the facilities that they would normally use. Certainly everyday professional resources would be quite inadequate to cope with the professional input that this programme utilised.

Regular modification of the programme did take place particularly during Stage II (see Ch. 3, pp. 57-61). However, it was one thing to let parents know that they could suggest and implement modifications to the programme and another for them to develop the confidence to suggest or ask for changes. Mittler and Schiefelbusch's writing (Mittler, 1975; Schiefelbusch, 1963) demonstrate the detailed understanding of the language of the intellectually handicapped that is required if teaching is to be effective. Snyder and McLean (1976) describe the distinctive features of children's language acquisition strategies. If these strategies are responsible for children's successful acquisition of language, then it would appear that an understanding of the conceptual framework underpinning these strategies is also required for successful teaching. This problem can only be overcome if a parent teaching programme can focus on the strategies which appear to be critical to the language development of the intellectually handicapped. Any modification suggested by parents to the original programme in this study focussed primarily on the "products" of language development. For example "I want my child to talk" was a prime parental aim. Any theoretical attempts to focus on children's strategies was observed to be "taking up valuable time", since the measure of improvement was increases in measured language age. However, when both parents and professionals had a similar, if not identical perception of a child's learning problem, then attention could and did focus on the child's learning strategies, rather than, or as well as, on the child's language output.

The continuing programme that Clunies Ross (1975) or Lovaas, Koegel, Simmons and Long, (1973) have written about would appear to provide the basis for the necessary correspondence between parent and professional. In these settings parents have time to develop confidence to suggest modifications to the teaching programme. Furthermore, they also will know that their ideas are likely to be implemented. This is reinforcing for parents.

Parents' perceptions of services even in an intervention programme are clearly different from those of the professionals. Throughout this programme a major issue for parents was the need for appropriate assessment procedures and for a means of guiding parent instruction, which in turn helped them to gauge their children's progress. Parents wanted accurate assessment and prescriptive teaching. It was clear that they did not want the one without the other. Whatever, the Psychologists' or Speech Therapists' or Counsellors' views of their traditional services, parents continued to emphasise that in the past, after assessment rarely had they been provided with information such as:

"Descriptions of my child's difficulties and/or deficit areas"

"Simple explanations of these deficit areas in relation to my child"

"Suggestions and plans as to the various teaching strategies that might help my child overcome these difficulties"

"Contact with a person or agencies who will *listen* to me at different stages in my child's development".

These views represent some parents' objectives for diagnostic services. There is little doubt that services for intellectually handicapped children provided by the Capital Territory Health Commission or the A.C.T. Schools Authority are not couched in these terms and despite the three years of this programme are unlikely to be. However, during discussions about the effectiveness of parents' teaching, there was regular face to face contact between parents and professionals. In addition an informal parent professional network was established that had not existed previously. This network helped to form the basis of groups' cohesion which in turn enabled parents to sustain their teaching during these three years.

Parents were involved in their child's language assessment in Stage I (see Ch. 3, p. 55). Parents did observe, wherever possible, the regular standardised assessment procedures O_2 to O_6, and they did present records of their daily teaching in the group training sessions. Videotapes of standardised language testing O_2 to O_5 and of parents' home based teaching were used as essential teaching materials during the group training sessions in Stage II. These video films also formed the basis of parents' discussions during Stage II about the effectiveness of their teaching. These videotapes provided much interest, and were regarded by parents as an efficient and most acceptable method of teaching.

Teaching parents about the distinctive feature of their children's language development proved to be a major task. This was not only because of the vastness of the topic, but also because of the tendency for the professionals involved to use linguistic and psycholinguistic terminology which parents did not necessarily understand. However, this topic and its influence on the writing of reports was discussed at length with parents during Stages I and II. The conclusions that were reached in these discussions were those which could be germane to any language teaching programme for the intellectually handicapped. Parents expressed their views during Stages II and III as to what were the distinctive features of language teaching for their children. These were features which could also be explicitly identified in simple reports, in the form that a child can or cannot perform at a particular level, along with the reasons as to why this is so. Essentially these distinctive features were:

(i) that understanding simple and then more complex commands and questions, can be achieved by the intellectually handicapped when a teaching programme comprises a series of small steps;

(ii) that these small steps begin with teaching effective attention-getting procedures and with establishing and then maintaining eye contact; this is then followed by the children learning signals from trained head shaking, eyebrow raising or frowning, to verbal responses such as "I don't understand". Teaching an intellectually handicapped child how to provide feedback that he/she is or is not understanding what is being said, may be determined by the speaker allowing the child sufficient time to reply. For example, response time for these children was often considerably longer than it was for normal children. A response time of at least 10 seconds after a question was not unusual;

(iii) that parents learned that facial, body and verbal cues and clues are given in the early stages of language teaching to help the child *always* get the right answer;

(iv) that children learned to respond either by gesture or by verbal responses to facial expressions such as eye contact, eyebrow raising, direction of gaze, head turning, smiling and the range of facial expressions which were used to convey interest, understanding or non comprehension;

(v) that parents learned that reinforcement was a signal (usually praise) to say that the right answer had been given;

(vi) that a child's motivation was a key to success, particularly in the development of expressive language and articulation skills;

(vii) that daily rehearsal of the same tasks was part of teaching and that this in turn enhanced a child's memory, particularly if consistent cues as in (iv) above were provided;

(viii) that each child works on the receptive and expressive language tasks which maintain his/her interest and, which also was likely to *extend* the child's language skills;

(ix) that regular testing and checking of a child's level of understanding and expression about classes of objects and events was part of the teaching programme;

(x) that evaluation of the linguistic characteristics associated with the intellectually handicapped must include descriptions of how these children process information; (as for example in (ii) above). This evaluation must try and identify the cues necessary for efficient language storage, retrieval and expression.

It is reasoned that if parents, and the many professionals involved, have a modicum of agreement on these ten points, then parents will be able to talk freely and openly about their children's language difficulties and development. Yet the professionals; teachers, counsellors and speech therapists, feel secure with their particular specialisations. If their knowledge and experience is in another area, then the particular difficulties of the intellectually handicapped may have low priority. In this situation, professionals can feel less secure about the specific and often detailed questions that parents of the intellectually handicapped ask. The professionals' apprehension, means, that parents become defensive and are considerably less willing to talk freely and openly. If therefore parents and professionals are to achieve some unison, a key factor would appear to be to employ professionals with detailed knowledge of the development of the intellectually handicapped and of the teaching programmes and strategies necessary for optimising that development.

The "helping services" of departments of health, education and welfare often appeared to parents of the intellectually handicapped as a "minefield of competing factions". Nevertheless, parents in this programme did feel that this "factionalism" could be minimised. The three years of professional and parent co-operation in this programme demonstrated that. Indeed, parents in this programme recognised that effective services depended on the working style and pragmatism of "a number of professionals". This was in a sense an article of faith; it was that if parents can work closely with professionals, (as the three years of this programme have demonstrated), then together they can shape and optimise service provision in the fields of health, education and welfare.

If comparable understanding by parents and professionals of the distinctive features of a language teaching programme is a priority, this is largely because it is a continuing problem that parents have in their contact with professionals. Underpinning this and analogous to it are parents' requests for **formalised** parent involvement. "Then we can stay in close touch with the teachers or therapists and develop confidence about our own abilities" remarked a parent of a 6 year old child with hydrocephaly. When this issue of formalising parent involvement in intervention teams or indeed in multidisciplinary health, education and welfare service teams was discussed during Stage III (see Ch. 3, p. 61) then five major reasons for the formal inclusion of parents were presented.

These were:

(i) that there are simply not enough professionally training and experienced staff to provide the necessary health and welfare care and educational and social interventions for these children. An obvious solution to this discrepancy is the use of parents or para-professionals to supplement the services provided by teachers, speech therapists, counsellors and social workers. Also the parent-child ratio presents an ideal teaching situation;

(ii) that parents spend so much more time with the child than any professional could hope to do. As such, the parent is apt to be more reinforcing to the child than most other adults. It is likely that when these teaching and reinforcing skills are developed the parent becomes not only the most available but also a most ideal teacher;

(iii) that behaviour directed and shaped in a clinic or office or indeed in a classroom is unlikely to generalise to other situations unless parents are involved. Furthermore, the adequacy of entire service delivery mechanisms, from the standardised assessment and clinical interview to some classroom settings, may well, inadvertently increase undesirable behaviour via inappropriate reinforcement programming. Successful service delivery may require modification of reinforcement patterns which exist in the children's natural social environment. When such changes in the environment prove to be necessary, then cost dictates engaging parents as primary behaviour change agents;

(iv) that direct parent involvement will help eliminate those repeated referrals which compound children and parents' insecurity. It will also facilitate appropriate questioning of the role that professional people play in this dilemma of repeated referrals;

(v) that there are parents who find it difficult to work effectively with their children (see above Ch. 6, p. 143). The inclusion of parents in a multidisciplinary team will help focus on finding alternative approaches for families with particular difficulties. The evidence of this research is that parents require as much individual programming as children (see above Ch. 6 and 7). Treating parents as a single, equal and homogeneous group is inappropriate. Parents require differing amounts of time with the professionals, not only because of their child's level of skills but also because of individual parental needs.

After three years of involvement in a home based intervention programme a fundamental and recurring question is whether parents really want to become involved. Does this programme provide irrefutable evidence of this? What has to be stressed again and again is that if teachers, speech therapists, counsellors and doctors are to be truly aware of the extra-ordinary problems that face families living with intellectually handicapped children, then nothing short of living with such children can sensitise them to these difficulties. To have parents involved in the provision of services will put the professionals closer to parents' needs and in so doing, will convince other parents of their own skills and endurance.

Answers to Research Questions

Some definitive answers have been given to the research questions and yet other answers are less conclusive. The principal answers to emerge were:

(i) that a structured behaviour modification programme was a most effective teaching method for developing intellectually handicapped children's receptive language skills over a period of three to six months, but that gains in receptive language skills were unlikely to be maintained over longer periods unless a controlled and monitored teaching procedure can become part of a family's domestic routine;

(ii) that a combination of developmental speech therapy and a structured behaviour modification programme was a most effective way of teaching expressive language skills, particularly if close attention was given to enhancing children's motivation to express their ideas, but that (as with receptive language skills) the initial gains were unlikely to be maintained unless the involved professionals **agree** on the expressive language goals and teaching procedures and were willing and able to give parents long term support;

(iii) that the provision of language manuals appears essential in a parent oriented language training programme but that the provision of the manuals **without** back up support is an ineffective means of intervention;

(iv) that children's sex, etiology and level of language development did not appear to effect the success of an intervention in developing children's receptive and expressive language skills, and in particular there was no evidence from this study that successful intervention is age specific; though chronological age was a guide in the assessment of children's language skills;

(v) that intellectually handicapped children's IQ scores were reliable and could be regarded as a guide to children's future development. However these IQ scores should not be regarded as fixed, immutable or unchanging;

(vi) that there was a close relationship between children's IQ scores and receptive language age scores but that the relationship between children's IQ scores and their expressive language age scores was less close, less related;

(vii) that it was possible to identify parents who were most able to teach their children language skills and those who were least able. This is not to say that those who were least able could not undertake such teaching, but rather that careful counselling and preparation to allay parents' frustration should be undertaken with these families before any language teaching commences. In particular, counselling with parents having difficulties should **emphasise** the role of structure in teaching and the importance of object specific play in children's language development;

(viii) that the majority of parents lacked a knowledge of the behavioural norms for their intellectually handicapped children and felt very uncertain when faced by professionals who they supposed understood these norms, but that these same parents at times had serious reservations about the skill and knowledge of some professionals, and that this often created uncertainty and unease in their relationships;

(ix) that these parents had great respect for their intellectually handicapped children and were personally so committed to providing optimum teaching and care that they were often tempted to participate in controversial therapy programmes, for which great claims were made. This may be because of the apparent dearth of options open to them, but also, was due to the absence of formalized parent involvement which in turn could result in closer relationship between parents and professionals working in the field;

(x) that individual case studies demonstrated the nature of the stimuli, reinforcement procedures and length of time necessary for these children to learn even the most simple language skill. It was the information in the case studies, relating to individual teaching procedures which was most relevant to parents and which in turn determined their motivation and perseverance in teaching their intellectually handicapped children.

Implications for Further Research

Many aspects of this longitudinal study require further research. In some respects the lists of further research activities could be endless, because of the lifelong nature of the task of bringing up and caring for an intellectually handicapped child. However, it is recommended that further research in the area of parents as language therapists concentrate on four areas. These are:

(i) Examination and identification of the factors influencing reinforcer effectiveness in language teaching. The use of praise when an intellectually handicapped child completes a task will in most instances strengthen the child's tendency to repeat that task under similar circumstances. However, parents realise that who gives the praise, what conditions precede the delivery of the praise, how many times it has to be repeated, and children's expectations concerning their parent's response are factors that may influence reinforcer effectiveness. In other words, the context in which supportive statements are made may be critical in determining whether they will function as effective reinforcers for the intellectually handicapped. Vivid illustrations of the problems to be encountered and the factors which are likely to determine the effectiveness of reinforcers are required. Certainly social reinforcement is one of the most complex forms of reinforcement and yet, it also is the form preferred by parents of the intellectually handicapped. Therefore, future research on this topic is required to provide clear illustrations of the difficulties encountered when parents, teachers or speech therapists try to discover whether a stimulus will function effectively as a reinforcer. Factors such as sex of the parent, teacher, or speech therapist, the influence of deprivation and satiation and people's roles are all likely to determine the effectiveness of social reinforcement. These factors need to be explicitly identified. There is also a need for these findings to be given some order, and some clear examples and illustrations, and answers to the problems which provoke parents or professionals to question the strength and flexibility of the social reinforcement paradigm;

(ii) The complexity of the language development of the intellectually handicapped means that if parents are to be involved in teaching their children then this complexity has to be reduced to understandable and manageable levels. Examples of this have been given above on p. 195. This research, and particularly the case study evidence in Chapter 7, illustrates that language acquisition for these intellectually handicapped children is an interactive process in which the child must function as an active participant. Exactly what strategies of comprehension and communication the intellectually handicapped use in this interactive process is not clear. If these strategies, (defined by Snyder and McLean, (1976) as "the entire repertoire of interactive behaviour and cognitive processes that enable a child to master the linguistic code of his culture . . .") can be identified, then they should be given some order and utilised in the teaching of receptive and expressive language skills. If research is able first to identify the strategies by which these children gather information and the environmental factors which influence the development of these strategies, then the research that must necessarily follow involves examining whether the intellectually handicapped can be taught these strategies under appropriate stimulus conditions;

(iii) There is always a danger that parents of intellectually handicapped children are typecast and as such are regarded as a homogeneous group as far as provision of services is concerned. The use of the PAAT in the research (see above Ch. 6, p. 143) identified parents who would be most or least likely to succeed in teaching their children. It is vital to identify the variables which determine whether parents are more able or less able to cope with having an intellectually handicapped child and/or are more able or less able to teach that child self-help skills and speech. If these variables can be identified, then the necessary health, education and welfare services can be adjusted accordingly. Cost effectiveness would also be enhanced. If "nothing short of living with such a child" highlights these parent/environmental variables then research would need to take this social anthropological form. No matter how advanced and sophisticated the language teaching programmes of the future are, if they do not, or cannot take account of parental and family differences then these programmes may be rendered quite ineffective in the short term.

198

Moreover there will be even less chance that the necessary parental perseverance over many years could ever be sustained.

(iv) The three years of this research have demonstrated that professionals in health, education and welfare can combine to provide comprehensive integrated services. The number of agencies inevitably involved with families of intellectually handicapped children suggests the necessity for co-ordination of services and liaison among professionals in the helping professions. Irvine (1979) argued for the primacy of parents as both co-ordinators of services and fully informed partners in all decisions affecting their handicapped children. There are far reaching implications in this proposition. Yet, since the conclusion of this "Parents as Language Therapists" research the professionals employed in the co-ordinated team have returned to their own departments to play their respective roles. Involving some parents of the intellectually handicapped as "named persons" (Special Educational Needs 1978) could keep the parent/client needs model to the fore. This research has conclusively demonstrated that this is feasible. In the future the formal involvement of parents in service provision has to be trialled so that their effectiveness as initiators and co-ordinators, as well as teachers of their children, can be evaluated.

If formal parent involvement is effective it would be a step towards focusing on needs from parents' points of view. In turn, formal parent involvement could provide that link which results in the establishment of genuine multidisciplinary health, eduction and welfare teams on a continuing basis. A resolution to this issue is imperative. Otherwise the fragmentation and division of health, education and welfare services may further discourage, if not put in jeopardy, parents' sustained commitment to optimising their children's future.

References

Abramowicz, H. K. and Richardson, S.A. Epidemiology of severe mental retardation in children: Community studies. *American Journal of Mental Deficiency*. 1975, *80*: 18-24.

Abramson, P. R., Grovink, M. J., Abramson, L.M., Sommers, D. Early diagnosis and intervention of retardation: A survey of parental reactions concerning the quality of services rendered. *Mental Retardation*, 1977, *15*(3): 28-31.

Ackerman, B. P. Children's understanding of definite descriptions: Pragmatic inferences to the speaker's intent. *Journal of Experimental Child Psychology*, 1979, *28*(1): 1-15.

Ainsworth, M. D. S. Social development in the first year of life: Maternal influences on infant-mother attachment. Unpublished paper presented at the Geoffrey Vickers Lecture, University of London, 1975.

Allen, G. Patterns of discovery in the genetics of mental deficiency. *American Journal of Mental deficiency*, 1959, *62*(5): 847-851.

Andrews, R. J. and Andrews, J. G. Early education for mentally retarded children. *Australian Journal of Mental Retardation*, 1974 *3*(1): 1-5.

Ansol, Occasional Papers No. 2. *Educating the handicapped child — segregation or integration?* Canberra. Australian National Social Sciences Library, 1976.

Baer, D. M. and Guess, D. Receptive training of adjectival inflections in verbal retardates. *Journal of Applied Behaviour Analysis*, 1971, *4*: 129-139.

Baer, D. M., Wolf, M. M. and Risley, T. R. Some current dimensions of applied behaviour analysis. *Journal of Applied Behaviour Analysis*, 1968, *1*: 91-97.

Baker, M. H. When the Down's syndrome baby is yours. *RN*, July, 1977 67-70.

Bandura, A. *Aggression: A social learning analysis*. Englewood Cliffs, New Jersey: Prentice Hall, 1973.

Bandura, A. Behaviour theory and the models of man. *American Psychologist*, 1974, *29*: 859-869.

Baroff, G. S. *Mental retardation: Nature, cause and management*. New York, John Wiley and Sons, 1974.

Bateson, M. C. The interpersonal context of infant vocalization. *Quarterly Progress Report, Research Laboratory of Electronics*, M.I.T., No. 100, 1971, 170-176.

Baumrind, D. Current patterns of parental authority. *Developmental Psychology*, 1971, *4*(1): Part 2, 103-104.

Bayley, M. *Mental handicap and community care*. London: Routledge and Kegan Paul, 1973.

Bayley, N. Development of mental abilities. In P.H. Mussen (Ed), *Carmichael's manual of child psychology, Vol. I.* New York: John Wiley and Sons, 1970.

Becker, W. C. *Parents and teachers*. Champaign, Illinois: Research Press, 1971.

Benassi, V. A. and Benassi, B. J. An approach to teaching behaviour modification principles to parents. *Rehabilitation Literature*, 1973, *34*: 134-136.

Bendebba, M. Contingencies management in home and school situations: A blueprint for the education of the "mildly retarded child". *Mental Retardation*, 1973, *11*: 34-37.

Berkowitz, B. P. and Graziano, A. M. Training parents as behaviour therapists: A review. *Behaviour Research and Therapy*, 1973, *10*: 297-318.

Berry, P. B. Elicited imitation of language: Some ESN(S) population characteristics. *Language and Speech*, 1976, *19*(4): 350-363.

Berry, P. B. and Foxen, T. Imitation and comprehension of language in severe subnormality. *Language — Speech*, 1975, *77*(4): 415-419.

Berry, P. B., Mathams, P. and Middleton, B. Patterns of interaction between a mother and her Down's syndrome child: A single case ethological study. *The Exceptional Child*, 1977, *24*(3): 156-164.

Bettison, S. Simple behaviour modification techniques as aids in teaching parents of autistic children child rearing principles. *Australian Journal of Mental Retardation,* 1973, *3*(3): 64-69.

Beveridge, M., Spencer, J. and Mittler, P. Language and social behaviour in severely educationally subnormal children. *British Journal of Social and Clinical Psychology,* 1978, *17*(1): 75-83.

Bice, H. *Group counselling with mothers of the cerebral palsied.* Chicago: National Society for Crippled Children and Adults, 1952.

Bidder, R. J., Bryant, G. and Gray, O. P. Benefits to Down's syndrome children through training their mothers. *Archives of Diseases in Childhood,* 1975, *50:* 383-386.

Bijou, S. W. and Werner, H. Vocabulary analysis in mentally deficient children. *American Journal of Mental Deficiency,* 1944, *48:* 364-366.

Bijou, S. W. and Werner, H. Language analysis in brain injured and non-brain injured mentally deficient children. *Journal of Genetic Psychology,* 1945, *66:* 239-254.

Bissell, J. S. *The cognitive effects of pre-school programs for disadvantaged children.* Washington, D.C.: National Institute of Child Health and Human Development, 1970.

Bloom, B. S. *Stability and change in human characteristics.* New York: John Wiley and Sons, 1964.

Bloom, L. *Language development: Form and function in emerging grammar.* Boston: M.I.T. Press, 1970.

Bloom, L. *One word at a time: The use of single-word utterances before syntax.* The Hague: Mouton, 1973.

Bloom, L. and Lahey, M. *Language development and language disorders.* New York, John Wiley and Sons. 1978.

Blount, W. R. Language and the more severely retarded: A review. *American Journal of Mental Deficiency,* 1968, *73:* 21-29.

Blount, W. R. Concept usage performance: Abstraction ability, number of referents, and item familiarity. *American Journal of Mental Deficiency,* 1971, *76:* 125-129.

Bock, R. D. *Multivariate statistical methods in behaviour research.* New York, McGraw Hill, 1975.

Bowerman, M. F. Discussion summary: Development of concepts underlying language. In. R. L. Schiefelbusch and L. L. Lloyd (Eds), *Language perspectives: Acquisition, retardation and intervention,* Baltimore: University Park Press, 1974.

Bowlby, J. The nature of the child's tie to his mother, *International Journal of Psychoanalysis,* 1958, *39:* 350-373.

Brewer, W. F. There is no convincing evidence for operant or classical conditioning in adult humans. In W. B. Weimer and D. S. Palermo, (Eds), *Cognition and the symbolic processes.* New York: Halsted Press, 1974.

Bricker, W. A. and Bricker, D. D. An early language training strategy. In R. L. Schiefelbusch and L. L. Lloyd, (Eds), *Language perspectives: Acquisition, retardation and intervention.* Baltimore: University Park Press, 1974.

Bronfenbrenner, U. *A report on longitudinal evaluations of pre-school programmes: Is early intervention effective?* Washington, D.C.: U.S. Department of Health, Education and Welfare, Office of Human Development, Children's Bureau, 1974.

Brown, D. G. *Behaviour modification in child and school mental health: An annotated bibliography on applications with parents and teachers.* Maryland: National Institute of Mental Health, 1972.

Brown, R. Development of the first language in the human species. *American Psychologist,* 1973, *28:* 97-106.

Bruner, J. S. Nature and uses of immaturity, *American Psychologist,* 1972, *27*(8): 687-708.

Bruner, J. S. The ontogenesis of speech acts. *Journal of Child Language,* 1975, *2:* 1-19.

Bruner, J. S., Jolly, A. and Sylva, K. (Eds), *Play: Its role in development and evaluation.* Harmondsworth: Penguin Books, 1976.

Brutten, M., Richardson, S. and Mangel, C. *Something's wrong with my child.* New York: Harcourt, Brace and Jovanovich, 1973.

Budoff, M. and Purseglove, E. M. Peabody picture vocabulary test performance of institutionalised mentally retarded adolescents. *American Journal of Mental Deficiency,* 1963, *67:* 756-760.

Burden, R. L. *Investigating maternal attitudes, an important aspect of the evaluation of an early intervention project with the mothers of severely handicapped children.* Proceedings of the British Psychological Society, University of Exeter, 1977.

Burgmeister, B., Blum, L. H. and Lorge, I. *Columbia mental maturity scale,* Harcourt, Brace and Jovanovich, New York, 1972.

202

Buscaglia, L. *The disabled and their parents: A counselling challenge.* Thorofore, New Jersey: Charles B. Slack, 1975.

Butterfield, W. H. and Parsons, R. Modelling and shaping by parents to develop chewing behaviour in their retarded child. *Journal of Behaviour Therapy and Experimental Psychiatry,* 1973, *4:* 285-287.

Carr, J.*Young children with Down's syndrome.* London: Butterworth, 1975.

Carrow, E. Assessment of speech and language in children. In J. E. McLean, D. E. Yoder and R. L. Schiefelbusch, *Language intervention with the retarded,* Baltimore, University Park Press, 1972.

Carrow-Woolfolk, E. Disordered language and its management. In E. L. Eagles (Ed), *Human communication and its disorders.* New York: Raven Press, 1975, 429-436.

Cartwright, D. The nature of group cohesiveness. In D. Cartwright and A. Zander (Eds), *Group dynamics.* New York: Harper and Row, 1968.

Centerwall, S. A. and Centerwall, W. R. A study of children with mongolism reared in the home compared to those reared away from home. *Pediatrics,* 1960, *25:* 678-685.

Chapman, R. S. and Miller, J. F. Early two and three word utterances: Does production precede comprehension? cited in R. L. Schiefelbusch and L. L. Lloyd, (Eds), *Language perspectives: Acquisition, retardation and intervention.* University Park Press, Baltimore, 1974.

Chazan, M. and Laing, A. F. *Young handicapped children: Services for parents of handicapped children under five.* Occasional paper, University of Swansea, 1978.

Chomsky, N. The general properties of language. In C. Millikan and F. Darley (Eds), *Brain mechanisms underlying speech and language.* New York, Grune and Stratton, 1967.

Clarke, A. D. B. and Clarke, A. M. Consistency and variability in the growth of human characteristics. In J. Sants and H. J. Butcher. *Developmental psychology, selected readings.* Harmondsworth, Penguin Books, 1975.

Clarke, A. M. and Clarke, A. D. B. *Mental deficiency: The changing outlook,* (3rd edition), London: Methuen, 1974.

Clarke, E. What's in a word? On the child's acquisition of semantics in his first language. In T. Moore (Ed), *Cognitive development and the acquisition of language.* New York: Academic Press, 1973, 65-110.

Clunies-Ross, G. G. A Model for early intervention with developmentally handicapped pre-schoolers. The children's centre at the Preston Institute of Technology. *Australian Journal of Mental Retardation,* 1976, *4*(4): 23-27.

Cochran, W. G. *Sampling techniques.* New York, John Wiley, 1963.

Cochran, W. G. and Cox, G. *Experimental design.* New York: John Wiley and Sons, 1957.

Constable, E., Ward, A., Jacobs, E., Shepherd, J., Drake-Brockman, C. *Parent education and assistance project. Final report; Evaluation.* Perth, University of Western Australia, 1979.

Cook, D. L. The Hawthorne effect in educational research. *Phi Delta Kappan,* 1962, *44:* 116-122.

Cooper, J., Moodley, M. and Reynell, J. Intervention programmes for pre-school children with delayed language development. A preliminary report. *British Journal of Disorders of Communication,* 1974, *9*(2): 81-91.

Cooper, J., Moodley, M. and Reynell, J. *Helping language development.* London: Edward Arnold, 1978.

Cooper, J., Moodley, M. and Reynell, J. The Developmental language programme. Results from a five year study. *British Journal of Disorders of Communication.* 1979, *14*(2): 57-69.

Crabtree, M. *The Houston test for language development, Pt. 1.* Houston Texas, Houston Test Company, 1969.

Cromer, R. F. Receptive language in the mentally retarded: Processes and diagnostic distinctions. In R. L. Schiefelbusch and L. L. Lloyd. *Language perspectives. Acquisition, retardation and intervention.* Baltimore University Park Press, 1974.

Cunningham, C. C. Parents as therapists and educators. In Study Group 8. *Behaviour modification with the severely retarded.* Manchester, Institute for Mental and Multiple Handicap. 1977.

Cunningham, C. C. and Jeffree, D. M. The organisation and structure of workshops for parents of mentally handicapped children. *Bulletin of the British Psychological Society,* 1975, *28:* 405-411.

Cunningham, C. C. and Sloper, P. Down's syndrome infants — A positive approach to parent and professional collaboration. *Health Visitor,* 1977, *50*(2): 32-37.

Cunningham, C. C. and Sloper, P. *Helping your handicapped baby.* London: Souvenir Press, 1978.

Decarie, T. *Intelligence and affectivity in early childhood.* New York: International Universities Press, 1965.

203

Dentler, R. A. and Mackler, B. The Porteus maze test as a predictor of functioning abilities of retarded children. *Journal of Consulting Psychology,* 1962, *26:* 50-55.

Dodd, B. Recognition and reproduction of words by down's syndrome and non down's syndrome retarded children. *American Journal of Mental Deficiency,* 1975, *80*(3): 306-311.

Downey, K. J. Parent's reasons for institutionalising severely mentally retarded children. *Journal of Health and Human Behaviour,* 1965, *6*(3): 147-155.

Drake-Brockman, C. *Parent education and assistance project. Final report. Project centre.* Perth. University of Western Australia, 1979.

Dunn, L. M. and Hottell, J. V. Peabody picture vocabulary test performance of trainable mentally retarded children. *American Journal of Mental Deficiency,* 1961, *65:* 448-452.

Edlund, C. V. Changing classroom behaviour of retarded children: Using reinforcers in the home environment and parents and teachers as trainers. *Mental Retardation,* 1971, *9:* 33-36.

Eisenson, J. Speech defects: Nature, causes and psychological concomitants in W. M. Cruickshank (Ed), *Psychology of exceptional children and youth.* New Jersey, Prentice-Hall, 1980.

Elkind, D. *A sympathetic understanding of the child: Birth to sixteen.* Boston. Allyn and Bacon, 1974.

Erwin, O. C. Comparison of articulation scores of children with cerebral palsy and mentally retarded children. *Cerebral Palsy, Review,* 1961, *22*(4): 10-11.

Estes, B. W., Curtin, M. E., DeBurger, R. and Deny, C. Relationships between the 1960 Stanford-Binet, 1937 Stanford-Binet, WISC, Raven and Draw-a-man. *Journal of Consulting Psychology,* 1961, *25:* 388-391.

Evans, D. The development of language abilities in mongols: A correlational study. *Journal of Consulting Psychology,* 1961, *21*(2): 103-117.

Evans, D., Hampson, M. The language of mongols. *British Journal of Disorders of Communications.* 1968, *3:* 171-181.

Eyeberg, S. M. and Johnson, M. S. Multiple assessment of behaviour modification with families: Effects of contingency contracting and order of treated problems. *Journal of Consulting and Clinical Psychology,* 1974, *42:* 594-606.

Fay, W. H. and Butler, B. V. Echolalia, IQ and the developmental dichotomy of speech and language systems. *Journal of Speech and Hearing Disorders,* 1968, *11:* 365-371.

Ferber, H., Keeley, S. M. and Shemberg, K. M. Training parents in behaviour modification: Outcome and problems encountered in a program after Patterson's work. *Behaviour Therapy,* 1974, *5:* 415-419.

Filler, J. W. Modifying maternal teaching style: Effects of task arrangement on the match-to-sample performance of retarded pre-school age children. *American Journal of Mental Deficiency,* 1976, *80*(6): 602-612.

Fink, W. T. and Bice Gray, K. J. The effects of two teaching strategies on the acquisition and recall of an academic task by moderately and severely retarded pre-school children. *Mental Retardation,* 1979, *17*(1): 8-12.

Flavell, J. H. *The developmental psychology of Jean Piaget.* New York: Van Nostrand Reinhold, 1963.

Flavell, J. H. Stage related properties of cognitive development. *Journal of Cognitive Psychology,* 1971, *2:* 421-453.

Frankenburg, W. K. and Dodds, J. B. *Denver development screening tests.* Ladnea Project and Publishing Foundation, 1970.

Fraser, C., Bellugi, U. and Brown, R. Control of grammar in imitation comprehension and production. *Journal of Verbal Learning and Verbal Behaviour,* 1963, *2:* 121-135.

Fredericks, H. D. B., Baldwin, V. L., McDonell, T. J., Hofmann, R. and Harten, J. Parents educate their trainable children. *Mental Retardation,* 1971, *9:* 24-26.

Freeman, S. W. and Thompson, C. L. Parent-child training for the mentally retarded. *Mental Retardation,* 1973, *11:* 8-10.

Fried, L. *The assessment of verbal communication skills of trainable mentally retarded children: A basic information quick test.* Los Angeles County Schools Office, Division of Special Education, L.A. 1977.

Friedlander, B. Z. Receptive language development in infancy: issues and problems. *Merrill-Palmer Quarterly,* 1970, *16:* 7-51.

Fries, C. C. *The structure of English.* New York: Harcourt Brace Jovanovich, 1952.

Frisch, S. A. and Schumaker, J. B. Training in generalised receptive prepositions in retarded children. *Journal of Applied Behaviour Analysis,* 1974, *7:* 611-621.

Fritsch, G., Fritsch, D. and Pechstein, J. Mothers of handicapped children and their loading capacity with therapeutic pedagogic duties: Comparison of connections between personality, self-image, social situation, attitude to the child and co-operation as co-therapist. *Montsschrift fur Kinderheilk unde,* 1976, *124*(5): 478-481.

Fromm, E. and Hartman, L. D. *Intelligence: A dynamic approach.* Garden City, New York: Doubleday, 1955.

Gajzago, C. and Prior, M. Two cases of "Recovery" in Kanner syndrome. *Archives of General Psychiatry, American Medical Association,* 1974, *31:* 264-268.

Gallagher, J. A. A comparison of brain injured and non brain injured mentally retarded children on several psychological variables. *Monograph, Social Research and Child Development,* 1957, *22:* No. 65.

Galloway, C. and Galloway, K. C. Parent classes in precise behaviour management. *Teaching Exceptional Children,* 1971, *3*(3): 120-128.

Gath, A. The impact of an abnormal child upon the parents. *British Journal of Psychiatry,* 1977, *130:* 405-410.

Gayton, W. F. and Walker, L. Down's syndrome: Informing the parents: A study of parental preferences. *American Journal of Diseases in Childhood,* 1974, *127:* 510-512.

Glass, G. V. and Stanley, J. C. *Statistical methods in education and psychology.* Englewood Cliffs, New Jersey: Prentice-Hall Inc., 1970.

Goertzen, S. M. Speech and the mentally retarded child. *American Journal of Mental Deficiency,* 1957, *62:* 244-253.

Goldberg, E. M. and Neill, J. E. *Social work in general practice.* London: Allen and Unwin, 1972.

Golden, D. A. and Davis, J. G. Counselling parents after the birth of an infant with Down's syndrome. *Children Today,* March-April, 1974 *3*(2): 7-11.

Golden, W., Hermine, M. and Pashayan, M. D. The effect of parental education on the eventual mental development of non-institutionalised children with Down's syndrome. *Journal of Pediatrics,* 1976, *89*(4): 603-605.

Goldfarb, W. Effects of early institutional care on adolescent personality. *Journal of Experimental Education,* 1943, *12:* 106-129.

Gorham, K. A. A lost generation of parents. *Exceptional Children,* 1975, *41:* 521-526.

Gould, J. Language development and non-verbal skills in severely mentally retarded children: an epidemiological study. *Journal of Mental Deficiency Research,* 1976, *20*(2): 129-146.

Gray, B. and Ryan, B. *A language program for the non-language child.* Champaign, Ill.: Research Press, 1973.

Green, A. C. H. and Soutter, G. B. The family and the young handicapped child: The importance of the right start. *Medical Journal of Australia,* 1977, *1:* 254-257.

Greenwald, A. G. Consequences of prejudice against the null hypothesis. *Pscyhological Bulletin,* 1975, *82:* 1-20.

Griffiths, R. *The abilities of babies.* London. University of London Press, 1964.

Grunewald, K. *The mentally retarded in Sweden.* Stockholm Division for Mental Retardation, National Board of Health and Welfare, 1969.

Guda, S. and Griffiths, B. C. Spoken language of adolescent retardates and its relation to intelligence, age and anxiety. *Child Development,* 1962, *33:* 489-498.

Guess, D. and Baer, D. M. An analysis of individual differences in generalisation between receptive and productive language in retarded children. *Journal of Applied Behaviour Analysis,* 1973, *6:* 311-329.

Guess, D., Sailor, W., Baer, D. M. *Functional speech and language training for the severely handicapped.* Lawrence, Kansas. H. and H. Enterprises. 1976.

Haley, J. (Ed), *Changing families.* New York: Grune and Stratton, 1971.

Hall, R. V. *Behaviour management series: Part I, the measurement of behaviour: Part II, basic principles: Part III, applications in school and home.* Merriman, Kansas: H. and H. Enterprises, 1971.

Hall, R. V., Axelrod, S., Tyler, L., Grief, E., Jones, F. C. and Robertson, R. Modifications of behaviour problems in the home with a parent as observer and experimenter. *Journal of Applied Behaviour Analysis,* 1972, *5:* 53-64.

Hall, R. V. and Broden, M. Behaviour changes in brain-injured children through social reinforcement. *Journal of Experimental Child Psychology,* 1967, *5:* 463-479.

Hanks, J. R. and Hanks, L. M. The physically handicapped in certain non-occidental societies. *Journal of Social Issues,* 1948, *4:* 11-20.

Hare, B. A. and Hare, J. M. *Teaching young handicapped children: A guide for pre-school and the primary grades.* New York: Grune and Stratton, 1977.

Haring, N. G. and Cohen, M. Using the developmental approach as a basis for planning different kinds of curricula for severely/profoundly handicapped persons. In *Educating the 24 hour retarded child.* Arlington T X: National Association for Retarded Citizens 1975.

Harrison, S. A review of research in speech and language development of the mentally retarded child. *American Journal of Mental Deficiency,* 1958, *63:* 236-240.

Harvey, A., Yep, B. and Sellin, D. Developmental achievement of trainable mentally retarded children. *Training School Bulletin,* 1966, *63:* 100-108.

Hawkins, R. P., Peterson, R. F., Schweid, E. and Bijou, S. W. Behaviour therapy in the home: amelioration of problem parent-child relations with the parent in a therapeutic role. *Journal of Experimental Child Psychology,* 1966, *4:* 99-107.

Heber, R., Dever, R. and Conroy, J. The influence of environmental and genetic variables on intellectual development. In H. J. Prehm, L. A. Hamerlynck and J. E. Crosson, (Eds), *Behavioural research in mental retardation.* Eugene, Oregon: School of Education, University of Oregon, 1968.

Heber, R., Garber, H., Harrington, S., Hoffman, C. and Falender, C. *Rehabilitation of families at risk for mental retardation: a progress report.* Madison: University of Wisconsin, December 1972.

Heifetz, L.J. Behaviour training for parents of retarded children: alternative formats based on instructional manuals. *American Journal of Mental Deficiency.* 1977, *82:* 194-203.

Heisler, V. *A handicapped child in the family: a guide for parents.* New York: Grune and Stratton, 1972.

Hemsley, R., Howlin, P., Berger, M., Hersov, L., Holbrook, D., Rutter, M. and Yule, W. Treating autistic children in a family context. In M. Rutter and E. Schopler (Eds), *Autism: A reappraisal of concepts and treatment,* London: Plenum Press, 1978.

Herbert, E.W. and Baer, D.A. Training parents as behaviour modifiers: Self recording of contingent attention. *Journal of Applied Behaviour Analysis,* 1972, *5:* 139-149.

Herbert, E.W., Pinkston, E.M., Hayden, M.L. Sajwaj, T., Pinkston, S., Cordua, G. and Jackson, C. Adverse effects of differential parental attention. *Journal of Applied Behaviour Analysis,* 1973, *6:* 15-30.

Herriot, P. *An introduction to the psychology of language.* London: Methuen, 1970.

Hewett, S. *The family and the handicapped child.* London: Allen and Unwin, 1970.

Hewson, S. *School-based parent's workshops — do they work?* In Proceedings of British Psychological Society Annual Conference, University of Exeter, April, 1977.

Hill, J. *Childrearing expectations of Navajo and Hopi parents of pre-schoolers.* Unpublished doctoral dissertation, Tempe, Arizona: Arizona State University, 1976.

Himelstein, R. Research with the Stanford-Binet Form L.M.: The first five years. *Psychological Bulletin.* 1966. *65:* 156-164.

Hindley, C.B. and Owen, C.F. The extent of individual changes in I.Q. for ages between six months and seventeen years in a British longitudinal sample. *Journal of Child Psychology and Psychiatry.* 1978. *19, 4:* 329-350.

Hirsch, I. and Walder, L.O. Training mothers in groups as reinforcement therapists for their own children. *Proceedings of the 77th Annual Convention of the American Psychological Association,* 1969, 561-563.

Ho, D. and White, D.T. Use of the full-range picture vocabulary test with the mentally retarded. *American Journal of Mental Deficiency,* 1963, *67:* 761-764.

Hofstaetter, P.R. The changing composition of intelligence: A study of the t technique. *Journal of Genetic Psychology,* 1954, *85:* 159-164.

Hofsten, C.V. and Lindhagen, K. Observations on the development of reaching for moving objects. *Journal of Experimental Child Psychology,* 1979, *28*(1): 158-173.

Honzik, M.P., MacFarlane, J.W. and Allen, L. The stability of mental test performance between two and eighteen years. In H. Mansinger (Ed), *Readings in Child Development.* New York: Holt, Rinehart and Winston, 1971.

Hood, P.N., Shank, K.H. and Williamson, D.B. Environmental factors in relation to the speech of cerebral palsied children. *Journal of Speech and Hearing Disorders,* 1948, *13:* 325-331.

Hopper, R. and Naremore, R.J. *Children's speech. A practical introduction to communication development.* New York: Harper and Row, 1978.

Hughes, A.S. Developmental physiotherapy for mentally handicapped babies. *Physiotherapy, 1971, 57:* 399-409.

Hume, A. The effectiveness of speech therapy for retarded children. Report to the Capital Territory Health Commission. Canberra 1978.

Hunter, M. and Shucman, H. *Early identification and treatment of the infant retardate and his family.* New York: The Shield Institute for Retarded Children, 1967.

Inhelder, B. *The diagnosis of reasoning in the mentally retarded.* New York: W.B. Stephens and John Day, 1968.

Irvine, J.W. On the delivery of special education services: The New England educational diagnostic centre. In *Australian Psychological Society: Proceedings of the Conference on Exceptional Children.* Newcastle, May, 1976.

Irvine, J.W. Decision making in special education: A plea for parent-professional partnerships, *Australian Journal of Special Education.* 1979, *3*(1): 23-24.

Jacobson, L.I., Bernal, G., and Lopez, G.N. Effects of behavioural training on the functioning of a profoundly retarded microcephalic teenager with cerebral palsy and without language or verbal comprehension. *Behaviour Research and Therapy,* 1973, *11*(1): 143-145.

Jaslow, R.I. and Stehman, V.A. (Co-Directors). *The decision to commit: a study of Detroit's retarded children.* Lansing, Michigan: Operations Research, Michigan Department of Mental Health, 1966.

Jeffree, D. M. and McConkey, R. Extending language through play. *Special Education: Forward Trends.* 1974, *1:* 13-18.

Jeffree, D.M. and McConkey, R. (Project Directors). *Parental involvement in facilitating the development of young mentally handicapped children.* A third progress report to the Department of Health and Social Security and the Department of Education and Science, London, August, 1976a.

Jeffree, D. and McConkey, R. *Let me speak.* London: Souvenir Press (E. & A.) Ltd., 1976b.

Jeffree, D.M., Wheldall, K. and Mittler, P. Facilitating two-word utterances in two Down's syndrome boys. *American Journal of Mental Deficiency,* 1972, *77*(3): 346-353.

Johns, N. Family reactions to the birth of a child with a congenital abnormality. *Medical Journal of Australia,* 1971, *1:* 277-280.

Johnson, A. An assessment of Mexican-American parent childrearing feelings and behaviours. Unpublished doctoral dissertation Tempe, Arizona: Arizona State University, 1975.

Johnson, M.A. *Teaching your retarded child: A parent's manual.* Melbourne: Cassell Australia, 1979.

Johnson, S.M. and Brown, R.A. Producing behaviour change in parents of disturbed children. *Journal of Child Psychology and Psychiatry,* 1969, *10:* 107-121.

Johnson, C.A. and Katz, R.C. Using parents as change agents for their children: a review. *Journal of Child Psychology and Psychiatry,* 1973, *14:* 181-200.

Johnson, J.T. and Olley, J.G. Behavioural comparisons of mongoloid and non mongoloid retarded persons: a review. *American Journal of Mental Deficiency,* 1971, 75(5): 546-559.

Kanner, L. Parent's feelings about retarded children. *American Journal of Mental Deficiency,* 1952, 57: 375-379.

Karlin, I.W. and Strazzulla, M. Speech and language problems in mentally deficient children. *Journal of Speech and Hearing Disorders,* 1952, *17:* 286-294.

Karlins, M. *Teaching retarded persons.* 14 television programmes presented by Minnesota Department of Public Welfare, St. Paul, Minnesota, U.S.A. 55101, 1972.

Karlsruher, A.E. The non-professional as a psychotherapeutic agent. *American Journal of Community Psychology,* 1974, *2:* 61-72.

Karnes, M.B. *Research and development program on pre-school disadvantaged children: final report.* Washington, D.C.: U.S. Office of Education, 1969.

Karnes, M.B. and Zehrback, R.R. Flexibility in getting parents involved in the school. *Teaching Exceptional Children,* 1972, *14*(5): 6-19.

Kazdin, A.E. Methodological and interpretive problems of single case experimental designs. *Journal of Consulting and Clinical Psychology,* 1978, *46*(4): 629-642.

Kazdin, A.E. Advances in child behaviour therapy. Applications and implications. *American Psychologist,* 1979, *34*(10): 981-987.

207

Keller, F.S. and Ribes-Inesta, E. (Eds), *Behaviour modification applications to education.* London, New York: Academic Press, 1974.

Kennedy, W.A., Van de Reit, V. and White, J.C. A normative sample of intelligence and achievement of negro elementary school children in the south-eastern United States. *Monographs of the Society for Research in Child Development.* 1963, *28:* No. 6.

Kent, L.R. with Klein, D., Folk, A. and Guenther, H. A language acquisition programme for the retarded. In J.E. McLean, D.E. Yoder, and R.L. Schiefelbusch. *Language Intervention with the Retarded. Developing strategies.* Baltimore, University Park Press, 1972.

Kerlinger, F.N. The first and second order factor structures of attitudes towards education. *American Educational Research Journal,* 1967, *4*(3): 191-205.

Kessler, J.W. Contributions of the mentally retarded toward a theory of cognitive development. In J. Hellmuth (Ed), *Cognitive studies Vol. I.* New York: Brunner Mazel, 1970.

Keys Smith, G. The handicapped child and society. The Mary Body Memorial Lecture for 1975. *St. Mark's Review, No. 84 — Caring for children.* Canberra, December, 1975, 3-17.

Kimber, A.A. and Porritt, D. *Parent reactions to "Parents As Therapists" programme to stimulate language development of intellectually handicapped children.* Clinical Evaluation Report No. 7, Capital Territory Health Commission, Mental Health Branch, November, 1976.

Kirk, S.A. *Early education of the mentally retarded.* Urbana, Ill.: University of Illinois Press, 1958.

Kirman, B. *Mental handicap: A brief guide.* London: Crosby, Lockwood, Staples, 1975.

Knobloch, H. and Pasamanick, B. Prediction from the assesment of neuromotor and intellectual status in infancy. In. H. Knobloch and B. Pasamanick, *Psychopathology of mental development.* New York: Grune and Stratton, 1967.

Kushlick, A. Social problems in mental subnormality. Ch. 5. In E. Miller, (Ed), *Foundations of child psychiatry.* Oxford Pergamon, 1968.

Latham, G. and Hofmeister, A. A mediated training program for parents of the pre-school mentally retarded. *Exceptional Children,* 1973, *39:* 472-473.

Lawrence, D. Counselling of retarded readers by non-professionals. *Educational Research,* 1972, *15*(1): 48-51.

Lazarus, A.A. Behaviour rehearsal vs non directive therapy vs advice in effecting behaviour change. *Behaviour Research and Therapy,* 1966, *4*(2): 209-212.

Lenneberg, E. H. Natural history of language. In F. Smith and G.A. Miller (Eds), *Genesis of language.* Cambridge, Mass: M.I.T. Press, 1966.

Lenneberg, E.H. *Biological foundations of language.* New York: John Wiley, 1967.

Lenneberg, E.H., Nichols, I.A. and Rosenberger, E.F. Primitive stages of language development in mongolism. *Disorders of communication. Vol. XLII: Research publications, A.R.N.M.D.* Baltimore: Williams and Wilkins, 1964.

Lerea, L. Assessing language development. *Journal of Speech Research.* 1958, *1:* 75-85.

Losen, S.M. and Diament, B. *Parent conferences in the schools.* Boston: Allyn and Bacon, 1978.

Lovaas, O.I., Berberich, J.P., Perloff, B.F. and Schaeffer, B. Acquisition of imitative speech by schizophrenic children. *Science,* 1966, *151:* 705-707.

Lovaas, O.I., Koegel, R., Simmons, J.Q. and Long, J.S. Some generalisation and follow-up measures on autistic children in behaviour therapy. *Journal of Applied Behaviour Analysis,* 1973, *6:* 131-166.

Luria, A.R. The directive function of speech in development and dissolution. In A. Bar-Adon and W. Leopold (Eds), *Child language.* Englewood Cliffs, New Jersey: Prentice-Hall, 1971.

Lustig, F.W. Some considerations concerning institutional placements of retarded children, *Medical Journal of Australia,* 1977, *1:* 257-260.

Lyle, J.G. The effect on an institutional environment upon the verbal development of imbecile children: (i) verbal intelligence. *Journal of Mental Deficiency Research,* 1959, *3:* 122-128.

Lyle, J.G. The effect of an institutional environment upon the verbal development of imbecile children: (ii) Speech and language. *Journal of Mental Deficiency Research,* 1960a, *4:* 1-13.

Lyle, J.G. Some factors affecting the speech development of imbecile children in an institution. *Journal of Child Psychology and Psychiatry,* 1960b, *1:* 121-129.

Lyle, J.G. Comparison of the language of normal and imbecile children. *Journal of Mental Deficiency Research,* 1961, *5:* 40-50.

McCall, R.B., Hogarth, P.S. and Hurlburt, N. Transitions in infant sensorimotor development and the prediction of childhood I.Q. *American Psychologist,* 1972, *27, 8:* 728-748.

McCarthy, D. Language development in children in L. Carmichael (Ed), *Manual of Child Psychology,* New York: John Wiley, 1965.

McCormack, E. *A handicapped child in the family,* London, Constable, 1978.

MacCubrey, J. Verbal operant conditioning with young institutionalised down's syndrome children. *American Journal of Mental Deficiency,* 1971, *75*(6): 696-701.

MacDonald, J.D., Blott, J.P., Gordon, K., Spiegel, B. and Hartmann, M. An experimental parent-assisted treatment program for pre-school language-delayed children. *Journal of Speech and Hearing Disorders,* 1974, *29, 4:* 394-415.

McIntire, R.W. *For love of children.* Los Angeles, California: C.R.M. Books, 1970.

Maratos, O. The origin and development of imitation in the first six months of life. Unpublished, Ph. D. Thesis, University of Geneva, 1973.

Marcus, L.M. Patterns of coping in families of psychotic children. *American Journal of Orthopsychiatry,* 1977, *47*(3): 388-399.

Mash, E.J. and Terdal, L. Modifications of mother-child interactions: playing with children. *Mental Retardation,* 1973, *11*(5): 44-49.

Mash, E.J., Lazere, R.L., Terdal, L. and Garner, A.M. Modification of mother-child interactions: a modelling approach for groups. *Child Study Journal,* 1973, *4:* 131-143.

Matheny, A.P. and Vernick, J. Parents of the mentally retarded child: emotionally overwhelmed or informationally deprived? *Journal of Pediatrics,* 1969, *74:* 953-959.

Melyn, M.A. and White, D.T. Mental and developmental milestones of non-institutionalised Down's Syndrome children. *Pediatrics,* 1973, *52*(4): 542-545.

Menyuk, P. *The acquisition and development of language.* Englewood Cliffs, New Jersey: Prentice-Hall, 1971.

Menyuk, P. The bases of language acquisition: Some questions. In E. Schopler and R.J. Reichler, (Eds.) *Psychopathology and child development: Research and treatment.* London, Plenum Press, 1976, 145-166.

Michaels, T. and Schuman, H. Observations of the psychodynamics of parents of retarded children. *American Journal of Mental Deficiency,* 1962, *66:* 568-572.

Milgram, N.A. Cognition and language in mental retardation: Distinctions and implications. In D.K. Routh (Ed). *The Experimental Psychology of Mental Retardation.* Chicago Aldine, 1973.

Miller, J.F. and Yoder, D.E. A syntax teaching program. In J.E. McLean, D.E. Yoder and R.L. Schiefelbusch (Eds), *Language intervention with the retarded: Developing strategies.* Baltimore: University Park Press, 1972a.

Miller, J.F. and Yoder, D.E. On developing the content for a language teaching programme. *Mental Retardation,* 1972b, *10*(2): 9-11.

Miller, S. J. and Sloane, H. N. The generalisation effects of parent training across stimulus settings. *Journal of Applied Behaviour Analysis,* 1976, *9*(3): 355-370.

Mira, M. Results of a behaviour modification training programme for parents and teachers. *Behaviour Research and Therapy,* 1970, *8:* 309-312.

Mittler, P. Language development and mental handicaps. In M. Rutter and J. A. M. Martin, (Eds), *Clinics in developmental medicine; The child with delayed speech.* No. 43. London: Heinemann, 1970.

Mittler, P. Language and communication. In A. M. Clarke and A. D. B. Clarke (Eds), *Mental deficiency: The changing outlook.* (3rd edition) London: Methuen, 1974.

Mittler, P. Language development in the mentally handicapped: An overview. In R. J. Andrews (Ed), *Language performance of exceptional children.* Fred and Eleanor Schonell Education Research Centre, University of Queensland, 1975.

Molony, H. Parental reactions to mental retardation. *Medical Journal of Australia,* April, 1971 *1*(17): 914-917.

Morehead, D. Early grammatical and semantic relations: Some implications for a general representational deficit in linguistically deviant children. *Language disorders in children,* 1972, (Special Issue No. 4).

Morehead, D. and Ingram, D. The development of base syntax in normal and linguistically deviant children. *Journal of Speech and Hearing Research,* 1973, *15:* 330-352.

Morse, P. A. The discrimination of speech and non-speech stimuli in early infancy. *Journal of Experimental Child Psychology.* 1972, *14:* 477-492.

Murphy, M. M. Comparison of developmental patterns of three diagnostic groups of middle grade and low grade mental defectives. *American Journal of Mental Deficiency,* 1956, *61:* 164-169.

Murray, M. A. Needs of parents of mentally retarded children. *American Journal of Mental Deficiency,* 1959, *63:* 164-169.

Myers, R. A couple that could, *Psychology Today,* 1978, *12*(6): 99-108.

Myers, P. A., and Warkany, S. F. Working with parents of children with profound developmental retardation: A group approach. *Clinical Pediatrics,* 1977, *16*(4): 367-370.

Myklebust, H. R. *Auditory disorders in children,* New York: Grune and Stratton, 1957.

Nelson, K. Structure and strategy in learning to talk. *Monograph of the Society for Research in Child Development,* 1973, *38* Nos 1. and 2.

O'Dell, S. Training parents in behaviour modification: a review. *Psychological Bulletin,* 1974, *81:* 418-433.

O'Kelly-Collard, M. Maternal linguistic environment of down's syndrome children. *The Australian Journal of Mental Retardation.* 1978, 5(4): 121-126.

Papania, N. A qualitative analysis of the vocabulary responses of institutionalised mentally handicapped children. *American Journal of Mental Deficiency,* 1953, *58:* 114-122.

Parks, R. M. Parental reactions to the birth of a handicapped child. *Health and Social Work,* August 1977, *2*(3): 51-66.

Patterson, G. R. *Families: applications of social learning to family life.* Champaign, Ill.: Research Press, 1971.

Patterson, G. R. and Gullion, M. E. *Living with children: New methods for parents and teachers.* Champaign, Ill.: Research Press, 1971.

Patterson, G.R., Cobb, J. A. and Rar, R. A. A social engineering technology for retraining the families of aggressive boys. In H. E. Adams and I. P. Unikel (Eds), *Georgia Symposium in Experimental Clinical Psychology,* 1973, *2.* Springfield, Ill.: Charles C. Thomas.

Payne, J. E. The deinstitutional backlash, *Mental Retardation,* 1976, *14:* pp. 43-45.

Peeters, T. Autistic children: Maternal attitudes and services. A cross cultural study. Unpublished MSc. thesis in the Faculty of Medicine, University of London, 1978.

Peine, H. A. and Munro, B. C. Behavioural management of parent training programs. *Psychological Records,* 1973, *73:* 459-466.

Piaget, J. *The language and thought of the child.* New York: Harcourt, Brace and Jovanovich, 1926.

Piaget, J. *Play, dreams and imitation in childhood.* London: Routledge and Kegan Paul, 1951.

Piaget, J. *The construction of reality in the child.* New York: Norton, 1954.

Piaget, J. Le language et les operations intellectuelles. In *Problemes de psycholinguistique: Symposium de l'association de psychologie scientifique de langue francaise.* Paris: Presses University France, 1963.

Piaget, J. *Biology and knowledge.* Chicago: University of Chicago Press, 1971.

Piaget, J. and Inhelder, B. *Mental imagery in the child.* New York: Basic Books, 1971.

Prechtl, H. F. R. The directed head turning response and allied movements of the human baby. *Behaviour,* 1958, *13:* 212-242.

Prior, M. Psycholinguistic disabilities of autistic and retarded children. *Journal of Mental Deficiency Research,* 1977, *21*(1): 37-45.

Pueschel, S. and Murphy, A. Counselling parents of infants with down's syndrome, *Postgraduate Medicine,* 1975, *58*(7): 21-24.

Rachlin, H. *Introduction to modern behaviourism.* (2nd edition). San Francisco: Freeman, 1976.

Ray, J. S. The family training centre: an experiment in normalisation. *Mental Retardation,* 1974, *12:* 12-13.

Raymond, M., Slaby, A. and Lieb, J. *The healing alliance.* New York: Norton, 1975.

Raymore, S. and McLean, J. E. A clinical program for carry-over of articulation therapy with retarded children. In J. E. McLean, D. E. Yoder and R. L. Schiefelbusch (Eds), *Language intervention with the retarded.* Baltimore: University Park Press, 1972.

Rees, R. J. *Parents as language therapists for intellectually handicapped children: Preliminary research report.* National Advisory Council for the Handicapped, Department of Social Security, Canberra, 1978.

Rees, S. J. *Social work face to face.* London: Edward Arnold, 1978.

Renfrew, C. E. *Speech disorders in children.* Oxford: Pergamon Press, 1972.

Revill, S. and Blunden, R. A home training service for pre-school developmentally handicapped children. *Behaviour Research and Therapy,* 1979, *17*(3): 207-214.

Reynell, J. K. A developmental approach to language disorders. *British Journal of Disorders of Communication,* 1969a, *4:* 33-37.

Reynell, J. K. *Reynell developmental language scales.* Slough: National Foundation for Educational Research, 1969b.

Reynell, J. K. Language handicaps in mentally retarded children. In A. D. B. Clarke and M. M. Lewis (Eds), *Learning speech and thought in the mentally retarded.* London: Butterworths, 1972.

Ribes-Inesta, E., Duran, L., Evans, B., Felix, G. and Sanchez, S. An experimental evaluation of tokens as conditioned reinforcers in retarded children. *Behaviour research and therapy,* 1973, *11* (1): 125-128.

Risley, R. T. and Wolf, M. M. Establishing functional speech in echolalic children. *Behaviour Research and Therapy,* 1967, *5:* 73-78.

Robinson, C. C. Application of Piagetian sensorimotor concepts to assessment and curriculum for severely handicapped children. *A A E S P H Review,* 1976,*1*(8): 5-10.

Roos, P. Parents and families of the mentally retarded. In J. M. Kauffman and J. S. Payne, *Mental retardation: Introduction and personal perspectives.* Columbus, Ohio. Charles E. Merrill, 1975, 339-359.

Rose, S. D. Group training of parents as behaviour modifiers. *Social Work.* (National Association of Social Workers), New York: 1974a *19:* 156-162.

Rose, S. D. Training parents in groups as behaviour modifiers of their mentally retarded children. *Journal of Behaviour Therapy and Experimental Psychiatry,* 1974b, *5:* 135-140.

Ross, D. M. and Ross, S. A. Cognitive training for the E.M.R. child: Language skills prerequisite to relevant-irrelevant discrimination tasks. *Mental Retardation.* 1979, *17* (1): 3-7.

Sailor, W. Reinforcement and generalisation of productive plural allomorphs in two retarded children. *Journal of Applied Behaviour Analysis,* 1971, *4*(4): 305-310.

Sailor, W. and Taman, T. Stimulus factors in the training of prepositional usage in three autistic children. *Journal of Applied Behaviour Analysis,* 1972, *5:* 183-190.

Sailor, W., Guess, D. and Baer, D. M. Functional language for verbally deficient children: An experimental program. *Mental Retardation,* June 1973, *11:* 27-35.

Sajwaj, T. Difficulties in the use of behavioural techniques by parents in changing child behaviour: Guides to success. *Journal of Nervous and Mental Diseases,* 1973, *156*(6): 395-403.

Salzinger, K., Feldman, R. S. and Portnoy, S. Training parents of brain-injured children in the use of operant conditioning procedures. *Behaviour Therapy,* 1970, *11:* 4-32.

Salzinger, S. K., Salzinger, K., Portnoy, S., Eckman, J., Bacon, P. N., Dentsch, M. and Zubin, J. Operant conditioning of continuous speech in children. *Child Development,* 1962, *33:* 683-695.

Sander, L. W., Stechler, G., Julia, M. and Burns, P. Early mother-infant interaction and 24 hour patterns of activity and sleep. *Journal of American Academy of Child Psychiatry,* 1970, *9:* 103-123.

Sandow, S. and Clarke, A. D. B. Home intervention with parents of severely subnormal pre-school children: An interim report. *Child Care, Health and Development,* 1978, *4:* 29-39.

Schiefelbusch, R. L. (Ed). Language studies in mentally retarded children. *Journal of Speech and Hearing Disorders,* Monograph Supplement No. 10, 1963.

Schild, S. Social Work Services. In R. Koch and J. C. Dobson, (Eds), *The mentally retarded child and his family: a multi-disciplinary handbook.* New York: Brunner-Mazel, 1971.

Schneider, B. and Vallon, J. A speech therapy program for mentally retarded children. *American Journal of Mental Deficiency,* 1954, *58:* 633-639.

Schneider, B. and Vallon, J. The results of a speech therapy program for mentally retarded children. *American Journal of Mental Deficiency,* 1955, *59:* 417-424.

Schumaker, J. and Sherman, J. A. Training generative verb usage by imitation and reinforcement procedures. *Journal of Applied Behaviour Analysis,* 1970, *3:* 273-287.

Seitz, S. and Riedel, G. Parent-child interactions as the therapy target. *Journal of Communication Disorders,* 1974, *7:* 295-304.

Semmel, M. I. and Dolley, D. G. Comprehension and imitation of sentences by down's syndrome children as a function of transformational complexity. *American Journal of Mental Deficiency,* 1971, *75*(6): 739-745.

Shearer, M. S. and Shearer, D. E. The Portage project: A model for early childhood education. *Exceptional Children,* 1972, *39:* 201-217.

Sheridan, M. D. *The developmental progress of infants and young children.* London. H.M.S.O. 1964.

Shipley, E., Smith, C. and Gleitman, L. A study of the acquisition of language free responses to commands. *Language.* 1969, *45*: 322-342.

Shontz, F. Reactions to crisis. *The Volta Review,* 1965, *67:* 364-370.

Sievers, D. J. A study to compare the performance of brain injured and non brain injured mentally retarded children on the differential language facility test. *American Journal of Mental Deficiency,* 1959, *63:* 839-847.

Simmons-Martin, A. A demonstration home approach with hearing impaired children. In E. Webster, (Ed), *Professional approaches with parents of handicapped children.* Springfield, Ill.: Charles C. Thomas, 1976.

Sinclair, H. Language acquisition and cognitive development. In T. Moore (Ed), *Cognitive development and the acquisition of language.* New York: Academic Press, 1973

Skeels, H. M. Adult status of children with contrasting early life experiences: A follow-up study. *Monographs of the Society for Research in Child Development,* 1966, Serial # 105, 31.

Skeels, H. M. and Dye, H. B. A study of the effects of differential stimulation on mentally retarded children. *Proceedings and Addresses of the American Association on Mental Deficiency,* 1939, *44:* 114-136.

Skelton, M. Areas of parental concern about retarded children. *Mental Retardation,* 1972, *10*(1): 38-41.

Skinner, B. F. *Verbal behaviour.* New York: Appleton Century Crofts, 1957.

Slobin, D. I. Grammatical transformations and sentence comprehension in childhood and adulthood. *Journal of Verbal Learning and Verbal Behaviour,* 1966, *5:* 219-227.

Slobin, D. I. Cognitive prerequisites for the development of grammar. In C. A. Ferguson and D. I. Slobin (Eds), *Studies of child language development.* New York: Rinehart and Winston, 1973.

Snyder, L. K. and McLean, J. E. Deficient acquisition strategies: A proposed conceptional framework for analysing severe language deficiency. *American Journal of Mental Deficiency,* 1976, *81*(4): 338-349.

Sommers, R. K. and Starkey, K. L. Dichotic verbal processing in down's syndrome children having qualitatively different speech and language skills. *American Journal of Mental Deficiency,* 1977, *82*(1): 44-53.

Sontag, L. W., Baker, C. T. and Nelson, V. C. Mental growth and personality development: A longitudinal study. *Monographs Society Research in Child Development,* 1958, *23.*

Sosne, J. B., Handleman, J. S. and Harris, S. L. Teaching spontaneous functional speech to autistic type children. *Mental Retardation* 1979, *17*(5): 241-245.

Sparrow, S. and Zigler, E. Evaluation of patterning treatment for retarded children. *American Journal of Pediatrics,* 1978, *62*(2): 137-150.

Special Educational Needs. Report of the committee of enquiry into the education of handicapped children and young people. London: HMSO, 1978.

Spitz, H. H. Field theory in mental deficiency. In N. R. Ellis (Ed), *Handbook of mental deficiency: Psychological theory and research.* London, New York: McGraw-Hill, 1963.

Spitz, R. A. Hospitalisation: An inquiry into the genesis of psychiatric conditions in early childhood. *Psychoanalytic Study of the Child,* 1945, *1:* 53-76.

Spitz, R. A. Anaclitic depression. *Psychoanalytic Study of the Child,* 1946, *2:* 313-342.

Spradlin, J. E. Language and communication of mental defectives. In N. R. Ellis (Ed), *Handbook of mental deficiency.* New York: McGraw-Hill, 1963a.

Spradlin, J. E. Assessment of speech and language of retarded children: The Parsons language sample. *Journal of Speech and Hearing Disorders, Monograph Supplement,* 1963b, *10:* 8-13.

Spreen, O. Language functions in mental retardation: A review. I. Language development, types of retardation, and intelligence level. *American Journal of Mental Deficiency,* 1965a, *69:* 482-494.

Spreen, O. Language functions in mental retardation: A review. II. Language in higher level performance. *American Journal of Mental Deficiency,* 1965b, *70:* 351-362.

Staats, A. W. *Learning language and cognition.* New York: Holt, Rinehart and Winston, 1968.

Staats, A. W. *Child learning, intelligence and personality.* New York: Harper and Row, 1971.

Stanford Research Institute. *Implementation of planned variation in Head-Start: Preliminary evaluation of planned variation in Head-Start according to follow-through approaches (1969-70).* Washington, D.C.: Office of Child Development, U.S. Department of Health, Education and Welfare, 1971a.

Stanford Research Institute. *Longitudinal evaluation of selected features of the national follow-through program.* Washington, D.C.: Office of Education, U.S. Department of Health, Education and Welfare, 1971b.

Stendler,C. B. Sixty years of child training practices. *Journal of Pediatrics,* 1950, *36:* 122-134.

Stinchfield, S. M. and Young, E. H. *Children with delayed or defective speech.* Stanford California, Stanford University Press, 1947.

Stone, H. The birth of a child with Down's syndrome: a medico-social study of thirty-one children and their families. *Scottish Medical Journal,* 1973, *18:* 182-187.

Stone, N. W. and Chesney, B. H. Attachment behaviours in handicapped infants. *Mental Retardation,* 1978, *16*(1): 8-12.

Stott, D. H. *The parent as a teacher: A guide for parents of children with learning difficulties.* London: University of London Press, 1972.

Strain, P. Increasing social play of severely retarded pre-schoolers with socio-dramatic activities. *Mental retardation,* 1975, *13*(6): 7-9.

Striefel, S. and Wetherby, B. Instruction following behaviour of a retarded child and its controlling stimuli. *Journal of Applied Behaviour Analysis,* 1973, *6*(4): 663-670.

Strom, R. D. Play and family development. *The Elementary School Journal,* 1974a, *74:* 359-368.

Strom, R. D. Observing parent-child play. *Theory into Practice,* 1974b, *13:* 287-295.

Strom, R. D. The merits of solitary play. *Childhood Education,* 1976, *52:* 149-152.

Strom, R. D. *Growing together: Parent and child development.* Monterey: Brooks/Cole. 1978.

Strom, R. D. and Johnson, A. Assessment for parent education. *Journal of Experimental Education,* 1978, *47*(1): 9-16.

Strom, R. D. and Slaughter, H. *The development of the parent as a teacher inventory: An instrument to measure the impact of parent education upon parent-child interaction variables.* Tempe: Arizona State University, 1976.

Strom, R. D. and Slaughter, H. Measurement of childrearing expectations using the parent as a teacher inventory, *Journal of Experimental Education,* 1978, *46*(4): pp 44-53.

Swann, W. and Mittler, P. Language abilities of ESN (s) pupils. *Special Education: Forward Trends,* 1976, *3:* 24-27.

T.A.C. The assessment clinic: Capital Territory Health Commission, Canberra, 1980.

Tavormina, J. B., Hampson, R. B. and Luscomb, R. L. Participant evaluations of the effectiveness of their parent counselling groups. *Mental Retardation,* 1976, *14*(6): 8-9.

Tawney, J. W. Acceleration of vocal behaviour in developmentally retarded children. *Education and Training of the Mentally Retarded.* 1974, *9:* 22-27.

Tein, R. G. Early Intervention via education programmes for parent-infants and young children with developmental delays and disabilities. *The Australian Journal of Mental Retardation.* 1977, *4*(6): 10-12.

Templin, M. *Certain language skills in children.* Minneapolis University of Minnesota Press, 160-162, 1967.

Terman, L. M. and Merrill, M. A. *Stanford Binet Intelligence Scale Form LM (Third Revision),* London: Harrap, 1961.

Tharp, R. and Wetzel, R. *Behaviour modification in the natural environment.* New York: Academic Press, 1970.

Tizard, B., Philips, J. and Plewis,I. Play in pre-school centres; I. Play measures and their relation to age, sex and IQ. *Journal of Child Psychology and Psychiatry,* 1976a, *17:* 251-264.

Tizard, B., Philips, J. and Plewis, I. Play in pre-school centres; II. Effects on play of the child's social class, and the educational orientation of the centre. *Journal of Child Psychology and Psychiatry,* 1976b, *17:* 265-274.

Tjossem, T. D. (Ed). *Intervention strategies for high risk infants and children.* Baltimore: University Park Press, 1976.

Torrance, E. P. Stimulation, enjoyment and originality in dyadic creativity. *Journal of Educational Psychology,* 1971, *62:* 45-48.

Tramontana, J. A review of research on behaviour modification in the home and school. *Educational Technology,* 1971, *11:* 61-64.

Trevarthen, C. Descriptive analyses of infant communicative behaviour. In H. R. Schaffer (Ed), *Studies in mother infant interaction,* London, Academic Press, 1977.

Tymchuk, A. J. Training parent therapists. *Mental Retardation,* October 1975, *13*(5): 19-22.

Ullman, L. P. and Kemp, C. H. Home intervention training programmes. In D. Harshburger and R. F. Maley, (Eds), *Behaviour analysis and systems analysis: an integrative approach to mental health.* Kalamazoo, Michigan: Behaviordelia, 1974.

Urban, A. An Early Intervention program in a remote area. *The Australian Journal of Mental Retardation,* 1978, *5*(3): 87-93.

Uzgiris, I. E. Patterns of vocal and gestural imitation in infants. In L. J. Stone, H. T. Smith and L. B. Murphy (Eds), *The competent infant,* Tavistock, London, 1974.

Uzgiris, U. C. and Hunt, J. McV. *Assessment in infancy: Ordinal scales of psychological development.* Urbana, B. Illinois, University of Illinois Press, 1975.

Vallett, R. E. *Modifying children's behaviour: A guide for parents and professionals.* Palo Alto, Calif.: Fearon, 1969.

Victorian Committee on Mental Retardation. Report to the Premier of Victoria, Melbourne, August 1977.

Vygotsky, L. S. *Thought and language.* Translated by E. Hanfmann and G. Vakar. New York: M.I.T. Press, 1962.

Vygotsky, L. S. Play: Its role in the mental development of the child, *Soviet Psychology,* 1966, *12*(6): 62-76. 76.

Wahler, R. G., Winkel, G., Peterson, R. and Morrison, D. Mothers as behaviour therapists for their own children. *Behaviour Research and Therapy,* 1969, *3:* 113-124.

Walder, L. O., Cohen, S. I., Breiter, D. E., Warman, F. C., Orne-Johnson, D. and Pavey, S. Behaviour therapy of children through their parents. In S. Golan and S. Eisdorfer, (Eds), *Handbook of community mental health.* New York: Appleton Century Crofts, 1971.

Walster, G. W. and Cleary, T. A. A proposal for a new editorial policy in the social sciences. *American Statistician,* 1970, *24:* 16-19.

Watson, G. Resistance to change. In W. G. Bennis, K. D. Benne and R. Chin, (Eds), *The planning of change.* New York: Holt, Rinehart and Winston, 1969.

Watson, L. S. *Child behaviour modification: A manual for teachers, nurses and parents.* Oxford: Pergamon, 1974.

Webster, E. (Ed). *Professional approaches with parents of handicapped children.* Springfield Ill.: Charles C. Thomas, 1976.

Webster, E. *Counselling with parents of handicapped children: Guidelines for improving communication.* New York: Grune and Stratton, 1977.

Wehman, P. and Marchant, J. A. Reducing multiple problem behaviours in a profoundly retarded child. *British Journal of Social and Clinical Psychology,* 1978, *17*(2): 149-152.

Weikart, D. P., Deloria, D., Lawsor, S. and Wiegerink, R. *Longitudinal results of the Ypsilanti Perry pre-school project.* Ypsilanti, Mi.: High/Scope Educational Research Foundation, 1970.

Weikart, D. P., Deloria, D. J. and Lawsor, S. Results of pre-school intervention project. In S. Ryan (Ed), *A report of longitudinal evaluation of pre-school programs.* (Vol. 1). Washington, D.C.: Department of Health, Education and Welfare, Publication No. (OND) 74-24, 1974, 125-134.

West, R., Kennedy, L. and Young, E. H. *The rehabilitation of speech* (Rev. ed.) New York, Harper, 1947.

Wheeler, A. J. and Sulzer, B. Operant training and generalization of a verbal response form in a speech-deficient child. *Journal of Applied Behaviour Analysis,* 1970, *3:* 139-147.

White, O. R. and Haring, N. G. *Exceptional teaching: A multi-media training package.* Columbus, Ohio: Charles E. Merrill, 1976.

Whitman, T. L., Zakaras, M. and Chandos, S. Effects of reinforcement and guidance procedures on instruction-following behaviour of severely retarded children. *Journal of Applied Behaviour Analysis* 1971. Vol. 4, 283-290.

Williams, J. L. and Jaffa, E. B. *Ice cream, poker chips and very goods: A behaviour modification manual for parents.* Maryland Book Exchange, College Park, Maryland, 1971.

Wing, L. *Autistic children: a guide for parents.* New York: Brunner-Mazel, 1972.

Wing, L. A study of language impairments in severely retarded children. In N. O'Connor, (Ed), *Language, cognitive deficits and retardation.* London: Butterworths, 1975.

Wolfe, W. G. A comprehensive evaluation of 50 cases of cerebral palsy. *Journal of Speech and Hearing Disorder.* 1950, *15:* 234-251.

Wolfensberger, W. *The principle of normalization in human services.* National Institute on Mental Retardation, Toronto: Leonard Crainford, 1977.

Wolpe, J. *Theme and variations: A behaviour therapy casebook.* Elmsford, New York: Pergamon Press, 1976.

Wood, N. E. Language development and language disorders: a compendium of lectures. *Monograph of the Society for Research in Child Development,* 1954, *25*(3): Lafayette, Indiana.

Wood, N. E. *Delayed speech and language development. Foundations of speech pathology series.* Englewood Cliffs, New Jersey: Prentice Hall, 1964.

Woodward, M. The behaviour of idiots interpreted by Piaget's theory of sensorimotor development. *British Journal of Educational Psychology,* 1959, *29:* 60-71.

World Health Organisation, *Organisation of services for the mentally retarded.* Fifteenth Report on the W.H.O. Expert Committee on Mental Health, World Health Organisation Technical Report, Series 392, Geneva, W.H.O. 1968.

Wright, J., Clayton, J., Edgar, C. L. Behaviour modification with low-level mental retardates. *Psychological Record,* 1970, *20:* 465-471.

Yoder, D. E. and Miller, J. F. What we may know and what we can do: Input toward a system. In J. E. McLean, D. E. Yoder and R. L. Schiefelbusch (Eds), *Developing strategies for language intervention.* New York: Holt, Rinehart and Winston, 1972.

York, R. and Williams, W. Curricula and ongoing assessment for individualised programming in the classroom. In R. York, P. Thorpe and R. Minisi (Eds), *Education of the severely and profoundly handicapped people,* Hightstown, N. J. Cohlen and N. Regional Resource Centre, 1977.

Yule, W. Treating autistic children in a family context. In M. Rutter and E. Schopler, (Eds), *Autism: A reappraisal of concepts and treatment.* London, Plenum Press, 1978.

Zeilberger, J., Sampden, S. and Sloane, H. Modification of a child's problem behaviour in the home with the mother as therapist. *Journal of Applied Behaviour Analysis,* 1968, *1:* 47-53.

Zifferblatt, C. E. Behaviour systems, In C. E. Thoresen (Ed), *Behaviour modification in education.* Seventy-Second Yearbook of National Society for Study of Education. Chicago, Illinois, University of Chicago Press, 1973.

Zigler, E. Developmental versus difference theories of mental retardation and the problems of motivation. *American Journal of Mental Deficiency,* 1969, *73:* 536-566.

Author Index

Subject Index

Appendix II

Preparatory, Receptive and Expressive Language Criterion Check Lists

Name of Child:

Task No.:	Task:	Mastery	Child's Score
		Correct response	
1.	Follows moving object with eyes		
2.	Stops movement in response to sound	"	
3.	Makes "startled" movement in response to sound	"	
4.	Turns toward the source of sound	"	
5.	Focuses on one object for 30 seconds	"	
6.	Moves mouth, chews food and swallows	"	
7.	Reaches for objects—shows eye-hand co-ordination	"	
8.	Points or gestures toward the objects he wants	"	
9.	Fixes eyes on and retrieves a rolling ball	"	
10.	Throws objects	"	
11.	Pushes and pulls objects	"	
12.	Uses hands to grasp objects (and shows preference)	"	
13.	Picks up objects in palm of hand	"	
14.	Picks up objects with fingers	"	
15.	Places objects such as cubes in containers	"	
16.	Places objects, e.g., pegs in holes	"	
17.	Places blocks to make vertical/horizontal structures	"	
18.	Turns pages of a book	"	
19.	Makes marks, e.g., spontaneous scribble using preferred hand	"	
20.	Makes controlled stroke with crayon or pencil	"	
21.	Sits still for up to one minute	"	
22.	Pays attention to your face for 30 seconds	"	
23.	Listens to music for one minute	"	
24.	Listens to spoken voice for one minute	"	
25.	Imitation skills—Crawling	"	
26.	Imitation skills—Clapping	"	
27.	Imitation skills—Waves "bye-bye"	"	
28.	Looks attentively at three random objects when presented individually	"	
29.	Looks attentively at five random objects when presented individually	"	
30.	Makes speech sounds—e.g., vocalizes two different sounds	"	

Raw Score Total: *30*   Child's Score:

APPENDIX IIb
Receptive Language Checklist
Profile at 0_2

Name of Child:

Task No.:	Task:	Mastery	Child's Score
1.	Commands	9/10	
2.	Commands	9/10	
3.	Pointing to objects named	9/10	
4.	Pointing to objects named	9/10	
5.	Use of objects that the child can point to	8/8	
6.	Looking for and finding concealed objects	8/8	
7.	Matching tasks (objects)	3/3	
8.	Matching tasks (pictures)	3/3	
9.	Searching for concealed objects	4/4	
10.	Placement of objects in relation to room parts	6/6	
12.	Pairing related objects	6/6	
13.	Finding concealed related objects	6/6	
14.	Colour sorting task	3/3	
15.	Commands and body/space awareness	10/10	
16.	Noun Vocabulary Group 11	9/10	
17.	Sorting exercise—concept big/little	10/10	
18.	Pointing to colour named	6/6	
19.	Commands involving verb and noun	6/6	
20.	Setting the table	6/6	
21.	Two stage commands	5/5	
22.	Recognizing and pointing to "big" objects	5/5	
23.	Counting tasks 1—5	5/5	
24.	Counting task with various objects—two five object sets	3/3	
25.	Counting task with various objects—three five object sets	3/3	
26.	Identifying an object by its colour (4/4)	4/4	
27.	Identifying an object by its colour (6/6)	6/6	
28.	Classification big/little objects (4/4)	4/4	
29.	Number of objects (1—5) on cards (4/4)	4/4	
30.	Number of objects (1—5) on cards (6/6)	6/6	
31.	Auditory/visual association exercises (3/3)	3/3	
32.	Auditory/visual association exercises (5/5)	5/5	
	Total possible:	194	

APPENDIX IIc
Expressive Language Checklist
Profile at 0₂

Name of Child:

Task No.:	Task:	Mastery	Child's Score
1.	Sounds for imitation	1/1	
2.	Sounds for imitation	3/3	
3.	Naming of body parts	6/8	
4.	Naming objects	8/10	
5.	Naming objects	8/10	
6.	Naming concealed objects	8/10	
7.	Sorting and naming colours	5/6	
8.	Naming concealed coloured blocks	5/6	
9.	Learing to count	5/5	
10	Possessive responses	4/4	
11.	Naming of objects in specific relationship to room parts	3/3	
12.	Naming of objects in specific relationship to room parts	3/3	
13.	Searching for and naming specific objects	6/8	
14.	Naming room parts in relationship to an object	5/6	
15.	Use of first verbs	3/3	
16.	Naming concealed objects	4/4	
17.	Naming objects in relation to a room part	3/4	
18.	Nouns using pictures	10/10	
19.	Naming concealed objects (Kim's game)	3/3	
20.	Naming concealed objects (Kim's game)	5/5	
21.	Counting objects	5/5	
22.	How many blocks?	5/5	
23.	Commands—use of verb plus noun	6/6	
24.	Commands—use of verb plus noun	6/6	
25.	Sentence response to the question "What can you see?" (objects)	8/10	
26.	Sentence response to the question "What can you see?"	8/10	
27.	Noun phrase and description	8/10	
28.	Verbal elaboration in response to pictures	8/10	
29.	Verb and Noun phrase *sentence* (response to pictures).	8/10	
30.	Verb and Noun phrase *conversation*	8/10	
	Total Possible:	194	

Appendix IV

Language Statements Presented to Parents During Stage 1

Language Development Programme

Language Statements Presented to Parents during Step I (June 1975)

Please tick the box which most adequately describes your child's capabilities.

LEVEL 1   LANGUAGE DEVELOPMENT

	YES	NO
My child is startled by sounds	☐	☐
My child is quietened by a soothing voice	☐	☐
My child anticipates feeding by opening mouth at seeing breast or bottle	☐	☐
My child makes vocalizations such as throat noises	☐	☐
My child shouts/cries for attention	☐	☐
My child searches for sounds with his eyes	☐	☐
My child sucks and bites objects and looks at them	☐	☐
My child smiles simultaneously	☐	☐
My child makes vocal social responses such as cooing	☐	☐
My child shakes head for "no"	☐	☐
My child vocalizes deliberately when communicating	☐	☐
My child makes vocal noises resembling speech sounds	☐	☐
My child babbles to himself in the mirror	☐	☐
My child makes single vowel sounds oh, uh, ah	☐	☐
My child screams with annoyance	☐	☐
My child chews solid food	☐	☐
My child listens to music	☐	☐
My child listens to babbling	☐	☐
My child listens to people talking	☐	☐
My child can tell strangers	☐	☐

LEVEL II   LANGUAGE DEVELOPMENT

	YES	NO
My child says connected syllables da-da-da	☐	☐
My child vocalizes when playing with toys	☐	☐
My child demonstrates affection to familiar people	☐	☐
My child turns immediately to father's and mother's voice across the room	☐	☐
My child claps hands in imitation	☐	☐
My child begins to imitate sounds after mother says them, e.g., ma-ma	☐	☐
My child understands "no no" and "bye bye" and responds to these	☐	☐
My child shouts to attract attention, listens and then shouts again	☐	☐
My child listens carefully to stop-watch ticking	☐	☐
My child uses facial and arm gestures to accompany vocalizations	☐	☐
My child knows and turns to his own name	☐	☐
My child communicates by pulling me to show me an object/situation	☐	☐
My child likes/listens to nursery rhymes	☐	☐
My child vocalizes his needs at the table	☐	☐
My child speaks one or two words	☐	☐
My child speaks up to four recognizable words	☐	☐
My child speaks up to six recognizable words and understands many more	☐	☐
My child understands and obeys simple commands	☐	☐

My child recognizes the names of up to five common objects when they are
    named   ☐   ☐

My child recognizes the names of up to ten common objects   ☐   ☐

My child enjoys listening to stories   ☐   ☐

My child has long babbled conversations to himself with many clear words   ☐   ☐

My child points to body parts when they are named   ☐   ☐

My child asks for food/drink (single word utterances)   ☐   ☐

My child says a few nursery rhymes   ☐   ☐

My child has up to *ten* words to express himself (mainly nouns)   ☐   ☐

My child names familiar objects for particular purposes   ☐   ☐

My child can name a number of objects in a picture correctly   ☐   ☐

My child puts two words together to make a phrase   ☐   ☐

My child listens attentively to stores for five minutes or more   ☐   ☐

My child communicates effectively by speaking in phrases or short sentences:
    "Look Mummy there"   ☐   ☐

My child has a vocabulary of 20 words   ☐   ☐

My child has a vocabulary of more than 20 words   ☐   ☐

My child identifies common pictures when they are named   ☐   ☐

My child matches common objects—ball/ball, car/car   ☐   ☐

My child matches common pictures   ☐   ☐

LEVEL IV   LANGUAGE DEVELOPMENT

My child lets us know (non-verbally) if he wants food or drink   ☐   ☐

My child understands simple questions—"What is that...?"   ☐   ☐

My child understands and correctly responds to simple requests   ☐   ☐

My child asks for food/drink   ☐   ☐

My child asks for toilet needs   ☐   ☐

My child understands two stage directions given consecutively, e.g., "Take your
    shoes off and put them in the cupboard."   ☐   ☐

My child talks to himself continually (using some jingle) during play   ☐   ☐

My child continually askes the names of objects   ☐   ☐

My child can name body parts   ☐   ☐

My child is capable of repeating words and phrases said to him   ☐   ☐

My child says a few nursery rhymes   ☐   ☐

My child knows his full name   ☐   ☐

My child knows his address   ☐   ☐

My child repeats words when excited   ☐   ☐

LEVEL V   LANGUAGE DEVELOPMENT

My child repeats whole phrases—"this a dog", "there a car"   ☐   ☐

My child verbalizes experiences—"go in car", "teddy in car"   ☐   ☐

My child asks "what", "where", "who" questions (but may still confuse them)   ☐   ☐

My child uses simple sentences—"me go out"   ☐   ☐

My child knows two nursery rhymes   ☐   ☐

My child can sing his nursery rhymes   ☐   ☐

My child begins to use plurals correctly   ☐   ☐

My child talks in monologues—concerned with immediate present   ☐   ☐

My child talks in monologues about make-believe stories   ☐   ☐

My child listens eagerly to stories and demands favorites over and over again   ☐   ☐

My child can tell his favorite story as he looks through his picture book   ☐   ☐

My child's speech is difficult to understand on some occasions ☐ ☐
My child still repeats words and parts of words when talking ☐ ☐
My child can make p (pie/pea/put) sounds correctly ☐ ☐
My child can make b (ball/bat/bee) sounds correctly ☐ ☐
My child can make m (mummy/man/me) sounds correctly ☐ ☐

LEVEL VI   LANGUAGE DEVELOPMENT

My child uses h (hat/hand/hair/horse) sounds correctly ☐ ☐
My child uses w (wheel/want/we) sounds correctly ☐ ☐
My child knows 2—3 colours ☐ ☐
My child knows 4—6 colours ☐ ☐
My child gives his age, sex, correctly ☐ ☐
My child can describe a recent event ☐ ☐
My child is *constantly* asking "why", "when", "how" questions ☐ ☐
My child tells stories (*connected* account of events!) ☐ ☐
My child is constantly asking the meaning of words ☐ ☐
My child constantly tries new words and phrases ☐ ☐
My child understands prepositional relationships—"in", "on", "under" ☐ ☐
My child uses personal pronouns (me, mine, his, her) correctly ☐ ☐
My child can make t (teddy/tea/take) sounds correctly ☐ ☐
My child can make d (day/dog/door) sounds correctly ☐ ☐
My child can make n/kn (no/never/knee) sounds correctly ☐ ☐
My child can make g (go/gone/gate) sounds correctly ☐ ☐
My child can follow and carry out *many* simple instructions ☐ ☐
My child can make ng (thing/ring/sing) sounds correctly ☐ ☐
My child can make y (yak/you/your) sounds correctly ☐ ☐

LEVEL VII   LANGUAGE DEVELOPMENT

My child acts out stories in detail ☐ ☐
My child gives his age and date of birth ☐ ☐
My child asks meanings of abstract words ☐ ☐
My child enjoys playing "mothers and fathers", "doctors and nurses" ☐ ☐
My child enjoys dressing up and participating in similar play situations with others ☐ ☐
My child talks regularly and fluently in play situations with other children ☐ ☐
My child can make f (fly/foot/fun) sounds correctly ☐ ☐
My child can make j (John/joke/jump) sounds correctly ☐ ☐
My child can make s (sit/Sam/sock) sounds correctly ☐ ☐
My child can make oh (on/onto) sounds correctly ☐ ☐
My child can make th (*thing*/*Th*ank you/*th*at) sounds correctly ☐ ☐
My child can make r (rug/rain/robot) sounds correctly ☐ ☐
My child can count to 5 ☐ ☐
My child can count to 10 ☐ ☐
My child can count to 20 or more ☐ ☐
My child's speech is fluent ☐ ☐